C0-AVH-589

# Group Work
# with the
# Frail Elderly

The *Social Work with Groups* series:

# Group Work
# with the
# Frail Elderly

Shura Saul
Guest Editor

Social Work with Groups
Volume 5, Number 2

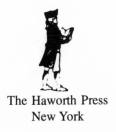

The Haworth Press
New York

Copyright © 1983 by The Haworth Press, Inc. All rights reserved. Copies of articles in the publication may be reproduced noncommercially for the purpose of educational or scientific advancement. Otherwise no part of this work may be reproduced or utilized in any form or by any means, electronic or mechanical, including photocopying, microfilm and recording, or by any information storage and retrieval system, without permission in writing from the publisher. Printed in the United States of America.

The Haworth Press, Inc., 28 East 22 Street, New York, NY 10010

**Library of Congress Cataloging in Publication Data**

Main entry under title:

Groupwork with the frail elderly.

    (Social work with groups ; v. 5, no. 2)
    Includes bibliographical references.
    1. Social work with the aged—Addresses, essays, lectures. 2. Social group work—Addresses, essays, lectures. I. Saul, Shura. II. Series: Social work with groups (Haworth Press) ; v. 5, no. 2.
HV45.S63      vol. 5, no. 2      361.4s            82-15600
[HV1451]                       [362.6'6]
ISBN 0-917724-77-1

# Group Work with the Frail Elderly

Social Work with Groups
Volume 5, Number 2

## CONTENTS

EDITORS

CATHERINE P. PAPELL, DSW, *Professor & Director, Direct Practice Division*
BEULAH ROTHMAN, DSW, *Professor Emeritus, Doctoral Program Adelphi University
School of Social Work, Garden City, Long Island, New York, 11530*


EDITORIAL ASSOCIATES

LOIS CZUGH, MA, *Adelphi University School of Social Work*
URANIA E. GLASSMAN, MA, MSW, *Adelphi University School of Social Work*


ADVISORY BOARD

ALBERT ALISSI, DSW, *University of Connecticut, School of Social Work, Greater
Hartford Campus, West Hartford*
HARVEY BERTCHER, DSW, *School of Social Work, The University of Michigan, Ann
Arbor*
LEONARD N. BROWN, DSW, *Graduate School of Social Work, Rutgers State
University*
MAX CASPER, MSW, *Syracuse University, School of Social Work*
HANS S. FALCK, PhD, *School of Social Work & Medical College of Virginia, Virginia
Commonwealth University, Richmond*
RONALD A. FELDMAN, PhD, *George Warren Brown School of Social Work,
Washington University, St. Louis, Missouri*
LOUISE A. FREY, MS, *Boston University School of Social Work*
MAEDA J. GALINSKY, PhD, *School of Social Work, University of North Carolina,
Chapel Hill*
JAMES GARLAND, MSSS, *Boston University School of Social Work*
CHARLES GARVIN, PhD, *School of Social Work, University of Michigan, Ann Arbor*
ALEX GITTERMAN, EdD, *Columbia University School of Social Work, New York*
PAUL H. GLASSER, PhD, *University of Texas at Arlington School of Social Work*
MARGARET E. HARTFORD, PhD, *Leonard Davis School of Gerontology, University of
Southern California, Los Angeles*
SUE HENRY, DSW, *Graduate School of Social Work, University of Denver*
CLARA KAISER, PhD, *Professor Emeritus, Columbia University School of Social Work,
New York*
ALAN F. KLEIN, MSW, JD, *Professor Emeritus, School of Social Welfare, State
University of New York at Albany*
RALPH L. KOLODNY, MSSS, *Boston University School of Social Work*
GISELLA KONOPKA, DSW, *Center for Youth Development & Research, University of
Minnesota, St. Paul*
NORMA C. LANG, PhD, *Faculty of Social Work, University of Toronto*
BARUCH LEVINE, PhD, *Jane Addams College of Social Work, University of Illinois,
Chicago; in private practice, Chicago*
HENRY W. MAIER, PhD, *Professor, School of Social Work, University of Washington,
Seattle*
RUTH R. MIDDLEMAN, EdD, *Raymond A. Kent School of Social Work, University of
Louisville, Kentucky*
HELEN NORTHERN, PhD, *School of Social Work, University of Southern California,
Los Angeles*
RUBY B. PERNELL, MSW, *School of Applied Social Sciences, Case Western
University, Cleveland*

HELEN PHILLIPS, DSW, *Professor Emeritus, School of Social Work, University of Pennsylvania, Philadelphia*

HERMAN RESNICK, PhD, *School of Social Work, Unviersity of Washington, Seattle*

SHELDON ROSE, PhD, *School of Social Work, University of Wisconsin, Madison*

LAWRENCE SHULMAN, EdD, *School of Social Work, University of British Columbia, Vancouver, Canada*

MARY LOUISE SOMERS, DSW, *Professor Emeritus, School of Social Service Administration, University of Chicago*

EMANUEL TROPP, MSSW, *Professor Emeritus, School of Social Work, Virginia Commonwealth University, Richmond*

ROBERT VINTER, PhD, *School of Social Work, University of Michigan, Ann Arbor*

CELIA B. WEISMAN, DSW, *Wurzweiler School of Social Work, Yeshiva University, New York*

GERTRUDE WILSON, MA, *Professor Emeritus, University of California, Berkeley*

## *IN MEMORIAM*

# WILLIAM SCHWARTZ
# 1916–1982

It is with a deep sense of loss that we mourn our friend and colleaugue, Bill Schwartz. As with so many others in this profession, he influenced us profoundly. We connect many of our deepest beliefs about group work with his ideas and scholarship. As editors, we shall particularly miss his cogent comments when he reviewed manuscripts for this journal as a member of its Advisory Board.

William Schwartz's theoretical contributions to the development of group work are unparelleled in this area. His unrelenting attention to the study of group work practice and to the professional activity of the worker, gave credence and validation to his theories. He introduced into social work the concept of mutual aid as an organizing principle in interaction processes.

He has, indeed, ''lent us a vision'' of the inherent strength of the group process and thus freed us as practitioners to fully risk ourselves in the service of others.

The following excerpt from a letter to Ruth Schwartz from Professor Derek Carter, a former student and now colleague in Northern Ireland, expresses what we feel our readers and contributors would want to say:

> part of Bill will live on in so many ways. He had much, much more still to contribute to social work and also to share more of his unpublished work with other practitioners and educators. There must be countless students who Bill touched during his teaching career who would wish to remember him in some formal way....I certainly would be willing to contribute to a memorial publication if other social workers who owe as much as I do to Bill would also be prepared to write papers in his honor.

© 1983 by The Haworth Press, Inc. All rights reserved.

*1*

Alex Gitterman and Lawrence Shulman have agreed to give leadership to the preparation of a special memorial issue of this journal dedicated to the continuity of ideas that were set down and into motion through William Schwartz's seminal work. It will carry, in Ruth Schwartz's words, "papers describing work now going on, that reflect Bill's ideas and how they get implemented day to day."

Colleagues wishing to participate in this undertaking may contact Drs. Gitterman and Schulman or the editors of this journal. We will keep our readers informed as the plan develops.

*Catherine P. Papell*
*Beulah Rothman*
*Co-Editors*

ALEX GITTERMAN, EdD
Associate Professor
Columbia University School of Social Work
622 West 113th Street
New York, NY 10025

LAWRENCE SCHULMAN, EdD
Professor
University of British Columbia School of Social Work
2075 Wesbrook Place
Vancouver, B.C., Canada V6T 1W5

# EDITORIAL

We are honored to publish this outstanding collection of papers concerned with the use of the social group work method with and in behalf of the frail elderly. The eloquence and knowledge of our guest editor, Shura Saul, her advisory committee and the authors that have been assembled give testimony to the broad commitments for our social group work colleagues and the contribution that group work can make to the fulfillment of life.

*CP*

*BR*

*GUEST EDITOR*

SHURA SAUL, EdD, CSW, *Educational Coordinator, Kingsbridge Heights Nursing Home; Adjunct Assistant Professor, Adelphi University School of Social Work, Brookdale Program; author of* The Right to be Different, *Chicago: Lionel Picheny Memorial Fund, 1962;* Aging: An Album of People Growing Old, *New York: John Wiley and Sons, Inc., 1974;* Sophia Moses Robinson: Woman of the 20th Century, *Garden City: Adelphi University Press, 1981; Consultant on Aging and Mental Health in this country and abroad.*

*ADVISORY COMMITTEE*

MARGARET HARTFORD, PhD, *Professor of Gerontology and Social Work, Leonard Davis School of Gerontology, University of Southern California*
LOUIS LOWY, PhD, *Professor, Boston University, School of Social Work*

© 1983 by The Haworth Press, Inc. All rights reserved.

# GUEST EDITORIAL

A myriad of stereotypes echo the term "frail elderly." Mental and physical impairments are often conceived in extremes of incompetence, rather than in degrees of capacity and limitation. The self and social image of persons thus categorized, becomes frozen. . . restricted to a very low expectation of individual behavior and to a potentially limited quality of life. There is often a social recoil from contact with our frail elderly: a recoil which may include professional helpers and caregivers, as well as the general public. There may be a tendency to avoid. . . a belief that a person having become old and frail has entered a downward spiral of mental, physical, social and emotional functioning.

Nothing could be further from the truth. Creative approaches leap beyond the double stigma of aging and frailty. They are geared to meet the dependencies; to support the frailties; and, thereby, to free each person to function at the highest point of individual capability.

These are some of the principles which underlie the approaches and programs described in this volume. All the papers speak to the recognition of frail elderly persons as human beings whose unique circumstances require special supports with the goal of establishing and maintaining a meaningful quality of life for each one. Whether the frailty is physical or mental, the psychosocial and emotional dimensions of the person remain open to supportive interventions.

Groups, in all their diversity, are viewed as creative approaches through which frail elderly persons may be reached for a variety of purposes; whose common denominators are affirmation of human identity, identification with others within a constructive social atmosphere, and enhancement of the life experience. Working with this vulnerable population, we are all required to rethink our own values, to recast our own assessment of meaningful living, to find our own rock-bottom concepts of purpose in life. We learn from them, again and again, about the vitality of human relationships, of the fruitfulness of mutual aid, of the productivity of caring and love. Frailty is a characteristic of the human condition. . . of people of all ages. We are each

© 1983 by The Haworth Press, Inc. All rights reserved.

of us in need of certain supports. The notion of "pure independence" is a chimerical one—no individual survives alone.

Our work with groups of frail elderly people as indeed, with all people, reminds us constantly of the ever present challenge to restore, within this automated society, our dedication to human need, human dignity, human life.

*Shura Saul*
*Educational Coordinator*
*Kingsbridge Heights Nursing Home*

# DEMOGRAPHIC CHANGE
# AND THE ELDERLY POPULATION

Mary J. Mayer

ABSTRACT. This paper reviews demographic trends and their implications for the growing population of elderly people, as well as their impact upon the total population of the nation. The nature and characteristics of frailty should be an area of major concern, as should the implications of frailty as related to service delivery. Although attention is being paid to the concept of frailty, no commonly accepted operational definition of frailty has as yet been developed.

A recent report by the Subcommittee on Human Services of the House Select Committee on Aging declares "Aging in America has changed. The meaning of the word, the size of the senior population, indeed the very process of aging itself—all have undergone radical transformations in the 20th century. So rapid and so pervasive are these changes that policy makers and public policies have barely kept up... Trends we see only dimly today, pressuring as they do almost every social and economic structure in our nation, will completely unfold in the near future...."

What are these changes and what are their implications?

First and foremost are the demographic changes. Since the turn of the century, the size of the nation's elderly population has increased steadily and dramatically. In 1900, there were only 3 million people over 65, who constituted 4 percent of the country's 76 million. By 1950, the number had quadrupled and represented 8 percent of the total. Thirty years later—that is, today—the number of elderly had doubled and its proportion had risen to 11 percent. Thus, while the total population had tripled since 1900, the elderly population increased eightfold. And the change continues. By the year 2020, it is estimated that every sixth American will be 65 or older.

Three basic demographic processes have contributed to this unprecedented

Mary J. Mayer is Director, Research and Planning, New York City Department of Aging.

[1]U.S. Congress, House Select Committee on Aging, Subcommittee on Human Services, "Future Directions for Aging Policy: A Human Service Model," p.2.

© 1983 by The Haworth Press, Inc. All rights reserved.

7

change: fertility, immigration and mortality. It is beyond the scope of this discussion to examine each of these factors in detail but mention should be made of the first two and must be made of the third. High fertility of the late 19th and early 20th centuries combined with the great waves of immigration during the same period produced the large cohorts that would later swell the ranks of the elderly. Then, as the birth rate fell during this century, these cohorts became proportionately more important in the total population.

Meanwhile, a third process was also making its significant contribution to the shape of the population. From ancient to modern times, an individual's average length of life has steadily increased. In this century, advances in medicine, nutrition, and sanitation have combined to make possible a startling jump in life expectancy. At the turn of the century in the United States, one could look forward on the average to a lifetime of 49.2 years. By 1978, this expectation had increased to 73.2 years.

If these figures are looked at another way, it can be said that one's earthly time allowance has rapidly shot up by the addition of nearly 25 years. Nothing comparable to it has been known before in the history of mankind. Although for some time it has been accepted that the body had been created to last a classic three score years and ten, until recently, there was all too evident proof that very few ever attained this and for a person to see his or her time out was exceptional. Literature refers to people being old at 40 in those days. Not so. Toil-worn and disease-marked by middle age, yes. But, apart from a minority whose lives extended as long as 70 or 80 years, most people were not involved in the aging process and seemed to have lived without thought or preparation for it. Life, because it was so often incomplete, operated on quite a different premise. In yesterday's world death was an accepted fact at any point in life; today it is seen as logically placed at the close of a long life.

Increased life expectancy has resulted not only in larger numbers of older people but also in significant changes in the age composition of this population. Three-fourths of the 7 million increase in the size of the older population anticipated between now and the year 2000 will be concentrated in the group 75 years of age and over. This differential growth, as Soldo points out,[1] is resulting in increasing proportions of those at the extremes of old age. Today nearly 4 out of every 10 persons over 65 are in the 75 and over cohort as compared with fewer than 3 out of 10 at the beginning of the century. By the year 2000, the figures will be pushing toward 5 out of 10. An even more dramatic increase is occurring in the proportion of the population 85 years of age and older: this group, only 4 percent of the elderly

---

[1]Soldo, Beth, "America's Elderly in the 1980's," Population Bulletin, p. 11.

population in 1900, is now 8 and is expected to soar to 12 percent in the next two decades.

One inevitable consequence of increased life expectancy is that for those who live to age 65, up to now a traditional retirement age, the post-working years are likely to last as long as childhood; if not longer. As former Commissioner on Aging Robert Benedict has noted, in effect a whole new generation is being added to the population. This fact, in turn, creates another demographic phenomenon that raises important questions of public policy as well as service issues. For, as more and more people live into their eighties and even nineties, more four generation families will exist. Grandparents who are themselves old will no longer be the oldest generation but will have even older parents still living.

However, increased life expectancy, though experienced by both sexes, has occurred differentially for men and women. Within the century, a curious and not wholly explained change occurred in the life expectancy of women. In the first half of the century, there was relatively little difference between the sexes in regard to survival rates. But after 1930, women began to survive longer than men. Based on death rates in 1975, average life expectancy at birth was 72.5 years. But males could expect to live 68.7 years while females could expect almost an additional 8 years, on an average of 76.5 years. This higher male mortality continues through the life span: men who reach age 65 have an average 13.7 years remaining; women over 4 years more—18.0 years. As a result, significant sex imbalance exists within the elderly population. Overall, six out of every 10 older Americans are women. With increasing age, the excess of females is even more pronounced. In 1979, among those 75 and older there were only 56 men for every 100 women. And the discrepancy is expected to widen further as the numbers of the "old-old" increase rapidly.

Two other demographic changes must be noted. The numbers of minority group elderly are increasing significantly, becoming a rapidly growing proportion of all elderly, especially in urban areas. Between now and the year 2000, it is estimated that the number of Black elderly will nearly double.

Finally, there are the living arrangements of older people. More a societal than demographic measure, nonetheless living arrangements are an important indicator in any discussion of the elderly population particularly because, as Soldo notes,[1] the living arrangements of the elderly are probably more varied than those of any other age group.

Twenty years ago, nearly half (46 percent) of those who were 65 years of age or older and had living children, lived with their children. By 1975, the

---

[1]Ibid, p. 26.

proportion had dropped to 18 percent. Older people in increasing numbers had begun to live independently of their younger relatives. The reasons for this dramatic change are several and all are complexly interwoven.

In this century, and especially following the second World War, as the nation became more urbanized and surburbanized and the population more mobile, there was a significant change in the structure of the family. The nuclear family household of parents and children became the dominant model. At the same time older people realized an improved economic status made possible by creation of the Social Security system. These factors, plus the ever present emphasis placed by Americans on independence, saw the formation of a significantly increased number of households headed by persons 65 years or older. Today, only a small fraction of the elderly live in the households of relatives or non-relatives or are institutionalized. About three-fourths of the elderly live in households in which they are either the head of the household or the spouse of the head. While the majority of these households consist of two or more persons, a significant, and increasing, proportion do not.

The most striking change in the living arrangements of the elderly in the period since World War II has been in the proportion of them living alone, especially women. Between 1950 and 1975, the rate of living alone for older men remained fairly constant (17 percent) but the proportion of women living alone skyrocketed from 25 to 41 percent.

Women and the "old-old" are much more likely than men or the "young-old to be living in something other than a conventional household of at least two persons. Between the ages of 65 and 74, only 12 percent of men are living alone compared with 35 percent of the women. By age 75 or older, the proportions living alone increase for both sexes but here again far more women (43 percent) are alone than are men (18 percent). Moreover women live with relatives to a significantly greater extent than do men. By age 75 or older, 18 percent of women are living in a relative's household compared with only 7 percent of the men, in general reflecting the fact that men remain married longer than do women.

What do these demographic phenomena imply? As pointed out earlier, not all the answers are in. But one fact seems clear. There is every likelihood that as the older population grows, two fairly distinct groups within it will be identifiable: those who tend to be relatively healthy and active and those who will be vulnerable and at risk because of greater impairment, poorer health or other deficits. In general, this latter group will tend to be found among the older elderly but not entirely. A significant proportion of those between the ages of 65 and 74 have been found to have characteristics of vulnerability.

Although continuing improvements in nutrition and developments in medical care has meant that on the average the health status of older people remains good for a long period of time, (only 14 percent see themselves in poor health) most older people do suffer from the presence of illness (usually chronic) and from some degree of functional impairment.

Almost half the people 65 and over are limited in activity because of one or more chronic conditions. About 13 percent of these are unable to carry out activities of daily living because their conditions affect their mobility. The prevalence of chronic illness and its impact on functional ability, moreover, means that older people require more medical help than is true for the younger population. The elderly visit doctors more frequently, are hospitalized more often and their stays are longer. The elderly also consume the majority of institutional long term care services. In general, health status declines and functional impairment increases with increasing age.

Older people also suffer from mental illness. The most common emotional disorders among the elderly are chronic anxiety and depression. Their rate of suicide is the highest of any age group. However, popular stereotype to the contrary, only 4 to 6 percent suffer from progressive deterioration of mental faculties.

Given the dramatic and sweeping changes occurring in the population and within the older population itself, which guarantee that as the aged population increases so will the size of the impaired population within it, there seems to be little question that the nature of frailty and the characteristics associated with it should be an area of major concern to policymakers, practitioners and researchers.

Although considerable attention has begun to be paid to the concept of frailty and the word is widely used in discussing the problems of older people remaining independently in the community, no commonly accepted operational definition of "frailty" has as yet been developed nor is there sufficient understanding of the complexity of the factors which determine frailty.

The one area of agreement is that frailty is multi-dimensional. In its 1977 Report to the President, The Federal Council on Aging saw frailty as the "accumulation of health, social, economic and environmental problems which impede. . .independent living."[1] However, there is less known about

---

[1]Federal Council on Aging, Annual Report to the President-1977, p. 35.

the implications of the dimensions of frailty as they relate to service delivery. If the needs of an important and growing segment of the elderly population are to be met, clearly more precise knowledge of the relationship of service needs to various patterns of the deficits that define frailty is essential for planners, policymakers, and practitioners.

## REFERENCES

Cantor, Marjorie and Menachem Daum, Extent and Correlates of Mental Health Vulnerability Among the Inner City Elderly Population. Paper presented at 27th Annual Meeting Gerontological Society, Portland, Oregon, October, 1974.

Federal Council on Aging, National Policy on the Frail Elderly. *Annual Report to the President-1977*. Washington, D.C. DHEW, 1978.

Federal Council on Aging, Public Policy and the Frail Elderly, a report prepared for USHEW, Office of Human Development Services, Washington D.C., December, 1978.

Johnson, Jeffrey L., Marjorie H. Cantor and Mary E. Collins, Multi-Dimensional Aspects of Frailty. Paper presented at 32nd Annual Meeting Gerontological Society, Washington, D.C. Nov. 1979.

Kovar, Mary Grace, "Elderly People: The Population 65 and over" in National Center for Health Statistics, Health, United States: 1976–1977, U.S.G.P.O., Washington, D.C., 1977.

Siegel, Jacob S., Prospective Trends in the Size and Structure of the Elderly Population, Impact of Mortality Trends and Some Implications, in Consequences of Changing U.S. Population: Demographics of Aging, Joint Hearings Before the Select Committees on Population and Aging, U.S. House of Representatives, U.S.G.P.O., Washington, D.C., 1978.

Soldo, Beth, America's Elderly in the 1980s, *Population Bulletin*, Vol. 35, No. 4 (Population Reference Bureau, Inc., Washington, D.C., 1980).

U.S. Bureau of the Census, Historial Statistics of the United States: Colonial Times to 1970, U.S.G.P.O., Washington, D.C.

———Current Population Reports, Series P-25, Nos. 311, 519, 614, 643, 704 and 970, U.S.G.P.O., Washington, D.C.

———Current Population Reports, Series P-20, No. 306, "Marital Status and Living Arrangements: March, 1976" U.S.G.P.O., Washington, D.C.

U.S. Congress, House Select Committee on Aging, Subcommittee on Human Services, Future Directions for Aging Policy: A Human Service Model, U.S.G.P.O., Washington, D.C. 1980

U.S. General Accounting Office, Home Health—The Need for a National Policy to Better Provide for the Elderly, U.S.G.P.O., Washington, D.C., 1980

# SOCIAL CARE FOR THE AGED
# IN THE UNITED STATES:
# ISSUES AND CHALLENGES

Marjorie H. Cantor

ABSTRACT. This paper reviews some of the impact of industrialization on the kinship structure and the shift in familial versus societal role re the elderly. Formal and informal networks of services and relationships are discussed: some needs and gaps in service identified. The role of women in filial responsibility within the modern family situation is noted and the need for increased supports identified. The author warns that both formal and informal systems—functioning complementary and optimally, are needed by the increasing number of elderly people.

The English poet John Donne, in the 17th century, perceptively noted that no man is an island unto himself and when the bell tolls for one it tolls for all. Acceptance of this concept of mutual interdependence has varied from society to society depending on its particular history, culture, and stage of economic development. A central theme of most cultures however has been the balance between the dependency and independency needs of individuals and society. In American pioneering days, out of necessity, the emphasis was on the ability of the individual to survive and prosper with a minimum of assistance from those around. Although the United States has long passed its frontier period, this ethos of independence and self-sufficiency still permeates our culture.

From the life cycle perspective there are, however, two significant stages in which society is more accepting of dependency needs—at the beginning and at the end. In the United States it is therefore considered appropriate for infants and children to be nurtured by parents as they are socialized into the culture. And again, as persons grow older and frailer society looks with greater tolerance on their needs for assistance and support.

However, in the case of old age, as the balance shifts from independence to dependency the potential for normative conflicts increases. Thus an older

Marjorie H. Cantor, DSW, is Brookdale Professor of Gerontology, Fordham University, Graduate School of Social Service.

© 1983 by The Haworth Press, Inc. All rights reserved.

person in the United States is caught in the dilemma between adherence to deeply rooted cultural norms of self-sufficiency and independence characteristic of adulthood and concrete needs for assistance as health, physical stamina, mobility and economic resources decline.

Some insight into how this value dilemma is mitigated in the United States, today, comes from an examination of the modern kinship structure and the relationship of the informal support system to formal organizations. The long standing pervasive myth of the elderly as isolated and abandoned without meaningful kin relationships has been destroyed by recent research (1, 5, 7, 13, 18, 19). Thus in urban industrial society the social support system of the elderly increasingly involves an amalgam of informal assistance provided by the family and significant others such as friends and neighbors and formal services offered by large scale organizations both governmental and voluntary, usually supported by public funds. Industrialization in America has been accompanied by an evolution in kinship structure from the traditional extended family to a more modified extended family. This modified family is characterized by a coalition of separately housed semi-autonomous nuclear families in a state of partial dependency who share with formal organizations the function of family (12). As a result there has been, in the United States, a shift in importance of the familial versus societal role regarding the elderly, particularly with respect to income maintenance, health and housing, but the family has by no means been supplanted by formal organizations. And nowhere is the role of family, friends and neighbors more crucial than in the provision of social care for the elderly (6).

What is a social care system and what are its main functions in the United States? A social care system can be viewed as a pattern of continuous or intermittent ties and interchanges of assistance that help an older person maintain their psychological, social and physical integrity over time. Consistency and availability of relationships and/or resources are required to meet social care needs whether of an on-going or time limited nature. Such a system is seen mainly as enabling an older person to fulfill three major needs: socialization, the carrying out of tasks of daily living and personal assistance during times of crisis or illness.

Older Americans perceive the informal network of kin (particularly spouse and children), friends and neighbors as the most appropriate source of social care in most situations and it is to this network that older people turn first and most frequently. Only when assistance from the informal system is unavailable or no longer able to absorb the burden of such care, is help sought from formal organizations. The social support system in the United States can therefore be categorized as hierarchal-compensatory, with kin as the first and preferred avenue of assistance followed next by friends/neighbors and lastly by government and other formal organizations.

One way of viewing the social care system in the United States is to envision an older person at the center of a series of concentric circles, each containing a different kind of support ranging from formal to informal. Usually these networks operate independently but at times they interact, as well as overlap.

In the outmost circle, furthest in social distance from the older person are the political entities, such as the United States Congress which determine the basic social policy and entitlements of older people. These entitlements impact significantly on the elderly's well-being particularly in the areas of income maintenance, health, housing safety and transportation. Somewhat close, though still far from playing a central role in daily life, are the governmental and voluntary agencies which carry out the economic and social policies and services mandated under such laws as the Social Security Act, Medicare and the Older Americans Act. All organizations in these two outer rings are clearly the formal part of the support system. Like all bureacratic organizations they attempt to function instrumentally and objectively according to an ideology of efficiency and rationality.

Still closer and standing somewhat between formal organizations and strictly informal networks of kin, friends and neighbors are the quasi-formal groups often called mediating forces. Examples of these are the postman, shopkeeper, church or neighborhood social group. Such groups or individuals resemble the informal network in their mode of operation yet they emanate from or are akin to formal organizations. Most important they often act as a bridge between the individual and broader society.

And finally closest to and, at the present time, most important as providers of social care are the informal caregivers—family (mainly spouse and children), neighbors and friends.

Research in New York City, and elsewhere discloses a pattern of reciprocal aid between generations, including emotional gratification, economic aid, child care, household management and health care (1, 3, 5, 6, 18, 19). The amount of help parents receive from children is related to the age of the parent and paucity of income suggesting that as older people become more vulnerable children respond with more assistance. Although our research in New York showed that the role of family as a support giver was strongest among the Hispanic population where the traditional extended family is more in evidence, White and Black elderly also have substantial informal support networks. And interestingly enough the extent of informal supports does not vary extensively by social class. Thus the family remains the prime caretaker of its older members in United States today (7, 8, 10).

Even more striking is the role of kin and significant others in providing services in the home when older people are sick or become frail. An analysis of two studies that sought to estimate the extent of current family responsibility to the functionally disabled suggests that between 60 and 85 percent of all such elderly receive a significant portion if not the entire assistance from family (11).

One final word about the formal social care system in the United States. Although there are available a wide array of formal services such as recreation and food programs, information and referral, legal services, employment programs, there is a striking paucity of home care and home health services as well as day care and respite provisions when compared with other industrialized countries. (For example in Sweden there are 923 home-help workers per 100,000 population as compared with 29 per 100,000 in U.S.A.). This lack is particularly noteworthy since it is estimated that one-fourth to one third of the elderly living in the community require home care services. Furthermore, about 8 to 10 percent of older community residents are considered to be as functionally impaired as the institutionalized elderly (1, 4, 14, 17). Lack of available home care, except from the informal system, stems in part from the original thrust of Medicare (the National Health Insurance program for the elderly) with its emphasis on acute care and its failure to address issues of chronic care. Although there is growing recognition of the need for home care services provided by the formal system there is yet no real acceptance of public responsibility in the provision of such services, except in the case of the poorest elderly without operable informal supports. The current economic climate is certainly a factor. But, I believe, more important is the lingering strength of the American ethos of self-sufficiency and rugged individualism. For many, social care is still seen as part of the welfare system and therefore equated with personal failure. This value premise can be found among persons of all generations, including the elderly.

But what of the future of social care? In any consideration of an appropriate balance between informal and formal components of a social care system, there are some important trends and issues which need consideration. Let me touch on a few.

1. The number of older people in the population relative to young adults is expected to continue to increase. Not only are the numbers of elderly expected to rise but in the United States and other western countries, the fastest growing segment of the elderly population are those over 75. (Thus projections suggest that in the United States between 1980 and 2010, the 85+ age cohort will increase 69%, the 75–84 cohort 40% while persons 65–74 in

the population will only increase 25%.) (15, 16) These are the very people who will need the greatest amount of assistance as they physically grow frailer and their economic well-being is further eroded by projected continuing inflation. Thus the need for social care will be more not less.

2. Yet women, the very group presently involved in providing most of the informal social care, are increasingly entering the labor market and remaining in it, even during the years of child rearing. The trend towards more working women is certainly influenced by the increase in divorce and single parent households. But working women are found as well in the traditional nuclear husband-wife household, where two wage earner families are one answer to inflation. Particularly significant is the continued rise in working among women aged 45–54, and 55–64, the very women who have traditionally contributed many hours to volunteer service and informal support of elderly parents.

However there is no indication that to-day's women, even those who work, are abandoning their filial responsibilities. Rather research suggests that these "women in the middle" (2) appear to be assuming multiple burdens of caring for their own families, and for aged parents, in addition to working. But the strain involved is considerable and some way must be found to lessen the burden if both younger and older families are not to suffer (1, 2, 3, 4, 9).

3. If the informal support system is a preferred mode of social care by older people and families provide so much of such care, serious consideration must be given to ways to assist family, friends, neighbors and other informal groups in their efforts? Support can come in the form of direct services, vouchers for service or cash allowances or a combination thereof. Some countries already have family allowances, tax rebates etc. In other places day care, respite and in-home care services help ease the burden of informal caregivers. In the United States, at present, there is a growing awareness that methods of assisting the informal networks are essential. But public policy does not yet reflect this awareness and there is as yet no coherent family policy.

4. Taking care of a frail dependent older person often involves considerable strain, particularly emotional for the informal caregiver. Special services geared to their needs, therefore, need to be considered. Several demonstrations are underway involving the formation of self-help groups of caregivers under the auspices of church or social agency. Through the sharing of experiences, knowledge about aging, knowledge of entitlements and connecting caregivers to available services, the burden is eased for the benefit of all concerned.

5. If in fact the informal social care system is considered to be a crucial part of the human service system, how do we insure that professionals recognize and support informal efforts? The question of proper interface between the formal and informal systems is crucial if the well-being of older people is to be advanced. To bring about a positive interface, training of the formal system in the value and importance of the informal must occur. Thus doctors, nurses, social workers etc. must learn to appreciate the role of family friends and neighbors and be willing to take the time to work with them and include them in service plans for older clients. Such interface probably involves radical changes in attitudes about professionalism, feelings of status and the importance of technical expertise. In the United States beginnings are being made in curriculum planning for new professionals and the retraining of those already on the job.

6. If we accept the premise that both informal and formal social care systems have unique value and that the welfare of older people is advanced by their cooperative efforts, we must make sure not to upset the delicate ecological balance between them. Thus the tendency to formalize the informal system, regulate, bureaucratize it, in our desires to strengthen and support poses a real and serious threat. How do you help mediating structures such as churches, and neighborhood groups play a role with the elderly without interfering with them? Even the granting of modest sums for start-up involves issues of accountability and regulation.

Similarly, is it better to provide assistance to informal caregivers through direct allowances or grants or is it better to make available more services such as homemakers etc. Should tax relief be given to older persons or their informal caregivers? In New York City, eligible older people were given money to procure their own homemakers without any real ongoing supervision. In some cases the frail older persons were victimized by the homemakers, in other situations homemakers failed to receive the employment benefits (i.e., Social Security) to which they were entitled. As a result, social agencies were called in to operate the program but such agency operation involves higher costs and more formal intervention. These are complex issues and solutions will differ depending on the mix of public and private social services in particular countries. But the basic problem of how to strengthen and assist the informal networks of family, friends, neighbors and local community groups without transferring them into formal entities and creatures of the state is applicable everywhere.

7. And finally in a climate of service retrenchment and economic constraint, we must reaffirm the role of community based publically supported social care services. Yes the informal social care system is valuable and has

PROPERTY OF WASHINGTON
SCHOOL OF PSYCHIATRY
LIBRARY

a unique role to play and is the system to which older people naturally turn first—but it cannot function unless there is a floor of comprehensive social care entitlements and services in place in the community. Particularly crucial are adequate home care services. Only with such a floor of services can we insure, on the one hand, that older persons without family, friends, or neighbors are adequately cared for. On the other, that assistance will be readily available when the need for care is beyond the capacity of the informal network. There is always the danger in periods of presumed limited resources and service reductions, such as are threatened in the United States, England, Germany at present, that the informal care system will be offered as a viable alternative for community based services. Such an approach would not only destroy the balance between informal and formal but it would certainly mean a serious reduction in care for older people. Only when both systems are in place and functioning optimumly, will the increasing numbers of elderly, in the future be assured the social care they need and desire.

## BIBLIOGRAPHY

1. Brody, Elaine, M. "The Aging of the Family," Annals, AAPSS, 438, July 1978.

2. Brody, Elaine, M. "Women in the Middle and Family Help to Older People." Paper presented at Symposium on the Family, sponsored by the Gerontological Society of America, 33rd Annual Meeting, San Diego, California, November 1980.

3. Brody, Elaine, M. "Women's Changing Roles, and Care of the Aging Family." *Aging: Agenda for the Eighties*, 1980.

4. Brody, Stanley, J. Comprehensive Health Care of the Elderly: An Analysis. *The Gerontologist*, Vol. 13, No.4, 1973, 412–418.

5. Cantor, M. "Life Space and the Social Support System of the Inner City Elderly of New York;" *The Gerontologist*, 1975, 15:23–27.

6. Cantor, M. "The Informal Support System: It's Relevance in the Lives of the Elderly:" in Borgotta and McCluskey (Eds) *Aging and Society*,Beverly Hills, London: Sage Publications, 1980.

7. Cantor, M. "The Informal Support System of New York's Inner City Elderly: Is Ethnicity a Factor?" in Gelfand and Kutzik (Eds), *Ethnicity and Aging*, New York, Springer Publishers 1979.

8. Cantor, M. "Neighbors and Friends: An Overlooked Resource in the Informal Support System." *Research in Aging*, Vol. III & Vol. IV, No.1–3 June 1979.

9. Cantor, M. "Caring for the Frail Elderly: Impact on Family, Friends, Neighbors." Paper presented at Symposium: Family Support of the Elderly, 33rd Annual Scientific Meeting, Gerontological Society of America, at San Diego, California, 1980.

10. Cantor, M. & Johnson, J. "The Informal Support System of the Familyless Elderly." Paper presented at Symposium: Informal Supports, Implications of Research for Practice and Policy, 31st Annual Scientific Meeting. Gerontological Society, Texas, 1978.

11. Congressional Budget Office, *Long Term Care*: Actuarial Cost Estimates, A CBO Technical Analysis (Washington, D.C., U.S. Government Printing Office, 1977) and U.S. Department of Health, Education and Welfare: 1978 HEW Task Force Report on Long Term Care, Washington, D.C., Office of the Secretary, Special Assistant to the Secretary of HEW, (Memorandum, 1978). Analyzed in Callahan, James et.al. "Responsibility of Families for their Severely Disabled Elderly," *Health Care Financing Review*, Winter 1980, pp. 29–48.

12. Litwak, Eugene. "Extended Kin Relations in an Industrial Democratic Society:" in *Social Structure and the Family*. Shanas and Streib, (Eds). Prentice-Hall, Inc.

13. *Future Directions for Aging Policy*: A Human Service Model, Subcommittee on Human Services of the Select Committee on Aging, U.S. House of Representatives, Ninety-Sixth Congress, May 1980, Comm. Pub. No.96–226.

14. National Retired Teachers Association, "Family Support Systems and the Aging: A Policy Report." *The American Family*.

15. United States General Accounting Office, "The Well-being of Older People in Cleveland, Ohio." HRD-77–70, Washington, D.C., U.S. Government Printing Office, 1977.

16. "Aging Groups in America, Recognizing Opportunities for Meeting their Needs," Appendix V, *Population Resource Center*, Project on Technology Adaptation and the Aging, New York, 1980.

17. "The Need for Long Term Care, Information and Issues," *Federal Council on the Aging*, U.S. Department of Health and Human Services, Office of Human Development Services, Washington, D.C. 20201, DHHS Publication No. (OHDS), 81–20704.

18. Shanes, Ethel. "Health Status of Older People: Cross National Implications." *American Journal of Public Health*, Vo. 64, No.3, 1974.

19. Shanes, Ethel. "The Social Myth as Hypothesis: The Case of the Family Relations of Older People." *The Gerontologist*, Vol. 19, No.1, 1979, pp. 3–9.

20. Sussman, Marvin B. & Burchinal, L. "Kin Family Network: Unhearalded Structure in Current Conceptualization of Family Functioning," Marriage and Family Living, 1962, 24: 231–240.

# SOCIAL GROUP WORK
# WITH VULNERABLE OLDER PERSONS:
# A THEORETICAL PERSPECTIVE

## Louis Lowy

ABSTRACT. This paper discusses the uses of social group work within the developmental model which looks at group life as a microcosm of the world. The author identifies the group as a modality for meeting differential needs of older persons. These needs are explored and some coincidence with the various stages of group development noted. The skills of the group worker are evoked on many levels—including that of making sound professional judgements regarding the appropriate use of the group for helping each individual. Groups for frail elderly persons may focus on one or more purposes.

## A Matter of Definition

A growing body of literature about the use of group methods for work with the aged is presently available. I am referring to Margaret Hartford's Chapter 33 in Birren and Sloan's *Handbook of Mental Health and Aging*[1] She writes,

> The uses of groupwork methods for work with the aged has occurred primarily in the past 35 years, reflecting the emergence of group services generally. The several strands of groupwork with the aged include: the services for the well elderly living in their own homes; homes of relatives, foster homes in retirement communities or other communal arrangements; group services for the frail elderly participating in day care centers, or out-patient therapeutic group sessions; and group services for the frail and dependent elderly who live in homes for the aged, hospitals for chronically ill or for the mentally ill, or long-term care facilities, nursing homes or convalescent homes."[2]

While there are a variety of group services for the elderly population, there is agreement that some of the same group methods focus on one or more

---

Louis Lowy, PhD, is a professor at Boston University, School of Social Work.
© 1983 by The Haworth Press, Inc. All rights reserved.

of the following purposes: the enhancement or rehabilitation of the person; improved interpersonal relationships between older people or between and among elderly and their families, relatives, friends or peers; problem-solving or achievement of tasks through collective action of elderly people; producing changes in the environment of participants in a group; designing action for changes of institutions or other organizations; creating changes in attitudes, values, social policies, programs and services by and for older people and the population in general.

Social group work is defined as one method of social work which places emphasis on maximizing group processes so that the group may become the instrument in which and through which the participating members may benefit, their interpersonal relationships may improve, and the participants may collaborate improving conditions in their environment. Social group-work is concerned with both, the growth and development of an individual person and with the development of interpersonal relationships to facilitate group processes for the achievement of collective goals.[3]

## Differential Needs of Older Persons

"Need" has a variety of meanings. It can signify a "condition marked by the lack of something requisite," (Webster) or "a requirement for survival, growth, health, social acceptance, etc."[4] To place "needs" on a scale of a minimal-optimal continuum is a useful device to categorize them, as Howard Y. McClusky has done, such as needs to cope, to express oneself, needs that are contributory and influence-exerting and those that give expression to meaning of one's existence, that gratify one's ego and allow for transcending it beyond the immediate time and place of life.[5]

Let us briefly review these needs within the life span of older people and then indicate how social groupwork can be instrumental in meeting these differential needs.

*Coping needs* come into play in order to meet fundamental survival concerns through adapting to changes associated with the aging process such as reductions in energy, and change in the social position of older people which are likely to result in reductions of income, health and functional ability of social affiliations, status and relationships. At the same time there is an expansion of disposable time and a greater freedom from certain role obligations. Coping with such changes requires adaptation because unless these coping needs are met successfully, there is little power left with which to meet the additional human needs. Taking Maslow's hierarchical concept, we can assert that opportunities for meeting survival needs through successful coping mechanisms—individually or socially supplied—are basic to meeting all other needs.

*Expressive needs* designate those strivings associated with fulfilling oneself by engaging in activities for their own sake and not necessarily to accomplish a task or reach a goal which can be designated as instrumental. In the later years, notably with more disposable time available and fewer work-role demands placed upon people (men and women), expressive needs can find greater potentialities for outlets, provided they have not been stifled too much during the preceding periods of the life cycle. Talents and interests dormant or alive can be stimulated to make the later years more expressively productive rather than merely instrumentally productive.

Expression of *contributory needs* are predicated on the assumption that people want to give to others, to their families, their friends and neighbors, to their "community," however defined. The blend of self-interest and altruistic interest in human beings is always fascinating; the extent of this blend constitutes a significant dimension of the human personality. Older persons certainly have the same need to share and negotiate the blending of "self and other interests" as have younger people. In addition, however, they have accumulated many life experiences, some digested, some undigested, some fragmented, some integrated—but they have a reservoir of contributions to be tapped by others, in the service to others—whether young, middle-aged or old. This is what Butler refers to as the "elder function" in a society, the task to leave a legacy and to contribute thereby to the heritage of civilization.[6]

We all need to exert some degree of *influence* on the factors impinging upon the conditions of our lives. Despite the impression that the degree of influence over our lives has appreciably diminished, we continue to strive to assert our powers of affecting the world we live in and it seems that without the illusion or reality of exerting some measure of influence, we would be unable even to meet our basic coping needs. As people grow older, their exertion of influence diminishes greatly, because they are relegated to inferior statuses, diminished positions of power in their social world as the results of ageist, discriminatory attitudes and practices in large parts of this world. And yet, as people grow older, they can exert influence over segments of their lives and their social world— individually and collectively—if they are consciously aware of the types of influences possible and if they associate with others, as the experiences of the "Gray Panthers" have quite effectively demonstrated. Older people want to continue to enjoy a sense of mastery and autonomy and exert some measure of control over certain aspects of their life-space, even those who are residents of total institutions.

All people at any stage in their lives need opportunities for expression of love and affection, for gratification of their ego-needs, for being assured that life has a purpose and meaning, At the later phases of the life cycle, this need seems even more pronounced than earlier where one is still more concerned with the todays and tomorrows than with the yesterdays, and when time to make up, time for restitution is diminishing. The *need for transcendence* rather than preoccupation with continued ego-involvement (as Peck phrases it)[7] appears to be a most profound need as one reaches the later years of one's life. What have I done with my life? (Erikson) Has it been invested with meaning? (Frankl) What legacy do I leave? (Butler)[8] To age successfully, indeed, means to come to terms with body-transcendence and to achieve a "sense of integrity" when completing the only life cycle available to any of us.

All older persons manage to meet those interrelated needs to varying extent, however their negotiating or coping abilities are affected by a number of variables, such as age, sex, race, ethnicity, position in the socio-economic structure, adaptive mechanisms to life tasks and crisis throughout their lifetime, state of health and functional ability, availability of social supports, informally and formally. Notably those older persons who have come to be defined as "frail elderly," those most vulnerable to debilitating conditions in the immediate environment, who have greater physical and emotional disabilities than their other contemporaries, those whose functional and coping abilities are more severely impaired and are therefore more dependent on psychological, physical and social support measures.[9]

What can social group work provide to elderly persons, particularly the more vulnerable, frail segment of this population in helping them meet this array of needs enumerated so far?

Hartford summarizes as follows:

> With the very old, the frail, dependent, handicapped, or ill, groups have been used for dealing with physical and emotional problems in outpatient or therapeutic services in the community or in institutions such as old age homes, nursing homes, and chronic and acute illness hospitals. In these groups the focus has been primarily on rehabilitation, restoration, or care and support. It is recognized that anxiety can be released and the emotions freed for use in healing of the individual through group discussion and activity, by playing out some of the fears, fantasies, and realities or by understanding better the nature of the problem. . . .
>
> . . . To some degree, groups of the frail elderly have also been used for activity, education, enhancement, and growth, just as with the well

elderly, except that their physical and/or mental capacities may be different and provide certain limitations.[10]

## *Developmental Model of Social Group Work*

A series of group work models have been identified in the literature.[11] Let me use the "Developmental Model" which I have participated in designing and which I have applied in my practice working with older persons. The "Developmental Model" looks at group-life as a "microcosm of the world" whereby experiences of members can be transferred to other situations in their lives. It emphasizes the dimensions of interpersonal closeness and distance and allows for gradual development of the individual to become a member with varying degrees of investments in the life of others. As a result, time processes become significant aspects of development which are marked as "phases of group life" with their own pace, as the goals of the group are based on the needs, aspirations and capabilities of its members and continue to satisfy these needs. Essential to guiding this process is the social group worker who must not only have understanding of the needs of individuals, of group formation and group development processes, but must also have skill in lending support on the one hand and making demands on the other, in order to keep up the tensions of interpersonal stimulation and hence, offer continued growth potential in negotiating closeness and distance of people to satisfy expressive, contributory, influence and ego-gratifying transcendental needs.[12]

## *Entry Phase: Group Formation*

During the entry stage when a group formation process gets underway, vulnerable older persons are most likely to be most apprehensive and psychological as well as physical distance are probably to be maintained at arms' lengths. To bring a few people together in greater physical proximity than heretofore is now the most important activity by the worker; people may not engage in interactional pursuits, nor take much notice of each other at first, but repeated contact may foster a breakdown of physical space barriers and lead to a lessening of physical, if not psychological distance.

Their coping needs are being addressed, as are their needs to exert some influence over their own life-space. To be near to somebody else may turn out to be useful to that "somebody else" and the older person has indeed contributed to others and even received from others, in turn. This points out the opportunities inherent in getting a group-formation process underway and meeting a number of needs of people without being yet involved in a "full-blown" group meeting. The group has not even begun to take off; indeed, it may never become a full-blown group with its attendant structural properties, such as norms, leadership, we-feelings, etc. In a nursing home, a number of residents during lunch hour sitting together at a table of four in the dining room can become engaged in such a tentative group formation process and find outlets for meeting expressive, contributory and influence needs, besides learning to cope with the demands of the staff by responding in novel fashions taught by a skilled social group worker!

This aggregate of older, frail people may remain an aggregate and not move beyond this pre-affiliative stage.[13] They may not want to become a group because their various needs can better be fulfilled by remaining "at a distance" to other peers and by establishing closer ties with their empathetic and skilled social worker. A bridge can be built that *may* lead to some degree of affiliation with other older (or younger) persons. Supportive networks *may* but need not evolve.[14] Now older people may find it more comfortable to take risks and to invest in others, to give and take, to listen and speak, to be passive and active. Testing of the situation becomes more feasible and desirable for some; yet others withdraw again for a while. The "minuet of two steps forward and three steps backward" gets a dress-rehearsal. There the social group worker is mindful of the opportunities and pitfalls, but also of the challenges to help assert the vulnerable, more isolated older person to come forth in a social encounter and learn to cope with power claims by others. Here are chances for meeting their needs for influencing others, for developing a sense of victory, of gaining a sense of autonomy, despite apparent waning powers, even a victory over the social worker in the office, or the nurse in the hospital, as one has practiced to assert one's powers over Mr. A or Mrs. B on the patient floor in a first gathering of the residents' group.

The "*power and control*" or "storming" stage in group development offers magnificent chances for testing, for trying out and trying on, for finding outlets for meeting coping, expressive, contributory and influence needs. This stage also provides people with an opportunity to release feelings which they otherwise would control to their disadvantage. Older persons who are afraid to get angry and are then immobilized by this fear have now a chance to observe others becoming angry and not being hurt by or punished for it. They are thus encouraged by the example of others via a mirror image to express this feeling instead of being thwarted by it. The example of others in the group who may be freer to express affection—being less fearful of rejection—may also help other elderly to experiment with expressive affection toward others more readily. This makes them more likely to receive more affection from others as well.

## Phase of Intimacy

When it happens that greater interpersonal closeness occurs over time as well as frequency of interpersonal encounters increases, then the *phase of intimacy* does appear, the phase usually referred to as the establishment of a "real group," characterized by the appearance of feelings of solidarity and group bonds and by the shaping of norms. In my experiences, this occurs more rarely among vulnerable older persons and, perhaps more importantly, it is not so relevant whether it does occur at all. To be sure certain aspects of the "intimacy stage" that replay family dynamics and demonstrate psychosocial closeness may not get played out at all when this phase is not reached, such as investment in love and affection, ambivalences, likes and dislikes of members and emotional attachments with other peers and the establishment of norms, the do's and don't's of group life. Needs for greater ego-gratification and affective expression may not find fulfillment to the extent desired by many a social worker. However, the energy of personal investment with attendant multiple losses, abandonment and accumulated frustrations when norm violations take place, may be too high a price to pay for the rewards of achieving the intimacy stage of the group. On the other hand, some people in the group may indeed proceed towards this phase and reap ego gratifications beyond their fondest dreams. Herein lies the assessment skill of the worker: to recognize how far to support the vision by assessing the older person's strengths and adaptive capacities to meet the demands of this stage. The worker must allow him/herself to be tested and re-tested and based on the result of these tests, formulate a "service contract," spelling out clearer mutual expectations between the older persons, the group members and him/herself.

Once a "group" has become established at this stage of development, the invariable group processes get played out: Who is on top and who is at the bottom? Who is close and who is distant? Who is accepted and who is rejected? Who adheres to the emerging norms and who does not? What are the sanctions for this? Feelings of dependency (upon the worker and/or peers) and independence (from worker and peers) get expressed more markedly now. To what extent can the vulnerable, older person tolerate "closeness" and norm-adherence during this stage as appreciable tolerance of closeness and norm conformity is expected? Research and demonstration reports indicate considerable success in mental hospitals and old age homes in working with deteriorated senile people suffering from chronic brain syndrome, to bring them into contact and communication through various forms of group therapy, though not necessarily of social group work.[15] Here the evidence is by no means in, though there is a body of practice-experience which confirms that hot-tempered exchanges, conflict-ridden argumentations provide many a ''frail'' older person with the essential juices to feel alive and to feel part of human interaction. Nowhere is this more essential than in institutional settings that value order and calm for organizational benefits over lively conflict and tension for continued human growth and vigor.[16]

Of particular relevance here is ''reminiscing.'' Not that reminiscing could not occur earlier in the group's development, but it is during the ''intimacy stage'' when reminiscing with other group members rather than merely with the worker is more frequent and can be utilized as a group rather than as a solo activity.

Much of the theoretical construct behind the value of reminiscing comes from Freud's discussion of the significance of early memories, both conscious and subconscious, as they influence later adaptations.[17] In social group work, however, only conscious material should be dealt with and the worker should avoid a consideration of the underlying causes of such behavior. As Pincus states:

> The worker's goal is to help the client make appropriate use of reminiscence. As always, the interventive plan should follow a careful assessment of the client's use of reminiscence... Simple empathic listening is important, but workers must go beyond this. They should accept the client and sensitize the relevant others in the person's situation (e.g., the members in the group) to the importance and functions of reminiscing and the need to encourage it in appropriate situations.[18]

And Ebersole states, ''The major reason to encourage reminiscing among a group of aged people is to produce or enhance a cohort effect.... They have little desire to affiliate with their own age group if they view it as devalued, out of step with the mainstream of life, or inadequate.''[19] And further: ''The second reason for group reminiscing with the aged is to increase opportunities for socialization by capitalizing on the exchange of early memories.''[20] In the early stages of group development the worker must be more active to insure that each participant is ''assured of time to talk and efforts must be made to emphasize, by re-statement, any expresion of feelings or concerns for other group members.''[21] If the group reaches ''intimacy stage,'' the group members will tend to do this for one another.

I could add here a third reason for group reminiscing: to help older people in general, but frail elderly in particular, to meet ego-transcending needs. The linking of the past with present and future can be facilitated through the appropriate use of reminiscing. Care must be taken when the material of the conscious past is painful and when "life review" leads to bringing up hurts and griefs without being able to cope with them. This is why corrective interventions not only by the worker but also by other group members are so vital and why the "stage of intimacy" lends itself to deal with meeting ego-transcending needs.

The final stage of group development is that of termination or *separation*. Many a group of older persons, particularly vulnerable older persons, may never reach a formal separation stage; they may, however, reach separation without ever going through an orderly process of any of the phases of group development. In fact, the likelihood that an aggregate of older persons will separate before becoming a fairly cohesive group is great, indeed. Peers move away from the neighborhood and join their families, some enter institutions (mostly permanently), others merely stop coming to the "group" and do not contribute to group building efforts, and others die. Separation and aloneness—if not loneliness—are frequent occurrences in the day-to-day lives of older people. And many have come to accept separation as a "normal loss." Here the social worker has to be particularly sensitive to avoid getting caught up in his/her own feelings, especially where the worker is much younger. The focus of the worker is to enable individuals to accept these losses without necessarily being able to replace them and yet, at the same time, to engage in grief work and to review earlier events, to recapitulate past experiences and to use reminiscing about relationships and events. When the aggregate had indeed become a group, then the support of others in doing grief work can be enlisted and separation losses become group rehearsals for future losses that are sure to occur. There we are dealing with "anticipatory grief work."[22] Exiting from the social world is as much part of the total human experience as is entering into it. And it is during the termination episodes when the needs for ego-transcendence can be most fully realized, as here the person is faced obliquely, surreptitiously or openly with the quest as to the meaning of life. Whether an answer will be sought depends on the way in which the worker (and other group members) utilize this opportunity to come to terms with this existential question. The most vulnerable elderly, whether at home or in a nursing care facility, as well as the least vulnerable elderly, face this ultimate question. Here spiritual feelings can be tapped and placed in the service of the ego to relate to the world of which one is a part. The interpersonal encounter is the instrument through which this relating can occur when the worker and his/her "coworkers," i.e., group members, engage in activities that facilitate coming to terms with a person's own finiteness on this earth.

*Activities in Social Group Work and the Worker*

Activities are means to ends; we can divide them into two major types: affective-expressive oriented and cognitive-instrumental oriented activities. The affective-expressive oriented activites include relating, empathizing, supporting, limiting, clarification of feelings around self and others, around things and conditions; the cognitive-instrumental activities include talking, discussing, programming, such as recreational, educational, creative and artistic, dramatic activities that respond to the interests, desires, motivation of older people at any stage of their emotional, mental and physical functional abilities.[23] These types of activities elicit coping abilities, a sense of mastery of the environment, problem-solving capacities, expression of self and affirmation of a person's sense of being here and now, with the possibility of transcending this moment and oneself.

The combination of affective-expressive and cognitive-instrumental activities is at the core of the social group work method as it is focussed on enhancing interpersonal relationships and collective activities for improving the quality of life. Even vulnerable, frail older people can experience the fruits of collective actions when they band together to achieve better nutrition in an institutional facility or more visible, humane caring of staff members in a hospital; they can indeed experience the results of collective endeavors when they actually obtain more reliable, homemaker services. But such collective action requires painstaking planning and preparatory efforts by a social worker who assesses carefully the strengths and weaknesses of the individuals, their readiness to risk themselves, their ability to affiliate with others, to take the "give and take" of group process and its inevitable conflicts of ranking and rating, of being accepted and rejected; in other words, the individuals' readiness and ability to become part of a group that will engage in collective action. On the other hand, the very engagement of taking collective action may create group solidarity and convince older people that they are less frail than assumed, less vulnerable than anticipated and the group encounter may strengthen them beyond expectation. Muscles that are not used tend to atrophy; energy that is not deployed tends to dissipate. The social worker's understanding and skill, appropriately deployed in the service of an achievable cause may bring forth latent strengths that stimulate the gratification of a plethora of coping, expressive, contributory, influencing and ego-gratifying transcending needs among seemingly or actual frail older persons who experience new heights of well-being never heretofore experienced because they were not appropriately stimulated. This is similar to "reality orientation" for treating confused elderly, which is predicated upon the theoretical notion that confused persons need constant direction, significant sensory involvement in the world around them and consistency in the approach to confront confused elderly with the "realities" of daily living.[24]

Through the "use of self," i.e., as an empathetic enabler, judicious mediator (broker) and as a focussed advocate for and with older people, the social group worker not only becomes a "role model," but also a reliable constant in the lives of older, vulnerable people who can be depended upon as much and as little as necessary to allow for maintaining their autonomy and to keep them engaged with others, including their family members, young and old. Since the final psychosocial task of achieving a "sense of integrity" is bound up with achieving ego-transcendence, the worker with older people, especially with those who experience greatest problems about this, has a defined mandate to create conditions that facilitate accomplishment of this task. The "group" in its varying stages of development can become an arena for this enterprise in the community as well as in an institution, though variables of each setting will affect the nature of the group process and its concomitant impact upon older people. Because interpersonal and group engagements may exert negative effects for some individuals that may lead to feelings of isolation, loneliness and rejection(e.g., when being scapegoated), the social worker must be particularly mindful of these potential problems and stresses and to know when and how to protect people from getting hurt, when exposure to group pressures are harmful to older persons and how to balance potential risks against potential benefits. This is precisely the type of judgments which social workers are expected to make. Making judgments are the hallmark of any profession for which professionals are held accountable by their peers and by the community. And using social group work in the service of older persons demands the value and attitude orientations and competency skills of a professional social worker.

## REFERENCES NOTES

1. Margaret E. Hartford, "The Use of Group Methods for Work with the Aged" in Birren, James E. and R. Bruce Sloane (eds.) *Handbook of Mental Health and Aging* (Englewood Cliffs, NJ: Prentice Hall, 1980), Chapter 33.

2. Ibid, p. 806.

3. Emanual Tropp, "Social Group Work: The Developmental Approach," pp. 1321-1327. William Schwartz, "Social Group Work: The Interactionist Approach," pp. 1327-1337. Paul H. Glasser and Charles D. Garvin, "Social Group Work; The Organizational and Environmental Approach" in *Encyclopedia of Social Work*, National Association of Social Workers, Washington, D.C., 1977.

4. Alfred J. Kahn, "The Function of Social Work in the Modern World," in *Issues in American Social Work* (NY: Columbia University Press, 1959), pp.3-12.

5. Howard Y. McClusky, "Education for Aging: The Scope and the Field and Perspective for the Future," pp. 324–331 in Stanley N. Grabowski and Mason W. Dean, *Learning for Aging* (Washington, D.C.: Adult Education Association, 1973).

6. Robert Butler, *Why Survive?* (NY: Harper and Row, Inc., 1975).

7. Robert Peck, "Psychological Developments in the Second Half of Life," in J.E. Anderson (ed.), *Psychological Aspects of Aging*(Washington, D.C.: A.P.A., 1956).

8. Erik H. Erickson, "Identity and the Life Cycle," in *Papers by E.E. Erickson* (NY: International Universities Press, 1959). Victor Frankl, *Man's Search for Meaning, 1962. Robert Butler, op. cit.*

9. Larry Branch, "When is an Elder 'Vulnerable'?," in *Harvard Medical Area Focus*, October 9, 1980.

10. Hartford, *op.cit.*, p. 814.

11. Catherine Papell and B. Rothman, "Social Group Work Models," in *Journal of Education for Social Work*, No. 2, Fall, 1966. James D. Garland and Ralph L. Kolodny, *The Treatment of Children Through Social Group Work: A Developmental Approach* (Boston: Charles River Books, 1981).

12. Louis Lowy, *Social Work with the Aging* (NY: Harper and Row, 1979), Chapter 12.

13. Garland and Kolodny, *op.cit.*

14. C. Crosby, "A Group Experience for Elderly Socially Isolated Widows" (Unpublished Master's Thesis, Los Angeles: University of Southern California, 1978).

15. Reichenfeld, H.F., Csapo, K.G., Carriere, L., and Gardner, R.C., "Evaluating the Effect of Activity Programs on a Geriatric Ward," in *Gerontologist*, 13 (3), pp. 305–310.

16. Mark Forman, "Conflict, Controversy and Confrontation in Group Work with Older Adults," in *Social Work*, 12, January 1967.

17. A.A. Brill, *The Basic Writings of Sigmund Freud* (NY: Random House, 1938).

18. Allen Pincus, "Reminiscence in Aging and its Implications for Social Work Practice," *Social Work*, 15 (4), October 1970, pp. 42–51.

19. Priscilla P. Ebersole, "Establishing Reminiscing Groups," in Irene M. Burnside, *Working with the Elderly: Group Processes and Techniques* (MA: Dubury Press, 1978), Chapter 15, p. 237.

20. Ibid, p. 239.

21. Ibid.

22. Avery Weisman, *On Dying and Denying* (NY: Behavioral Publications, 1970).

23. I.M. Burnside, *Working with the Elderly: Group Processes and Techniques.*

24. Lucille R. Taulbee, "Reality Orientation: A Therapeutic Group Activity for Elderly Persons," in I.M. Burnside, *Working with the Elderly: Group Processes and Techniques* (MA: Dubury Press, 1978), Chapter 13.

# DIFFERENTIAL USE OF GROUPS
# IN MAINSTREAMING
# THE HANDICAPPED ELDERLY

Harriette Friedlander

ABSTRACT. This article describes the experience of Selfhelp Community Services in establishing a day center for the physically frail handicapped aged. Through the use of groups and other support services, a program for the isolated homebound is developed and maintained. Goals of the program include prevention of premature institutionalization, restoration of socialization skills, enhancement of individual self esteem, and respite for families. The evolution of the program from its beginning as a self standing center to its present structure as an integrated service in a multipurpose senior center is described.

From the minute you walk in you sense that there is something different about this senior center. A group of handicapped older people most of them in wheelchairs, is seen functioning side by side with the normal mix of healthy and not so healthy older adults that attend the many similar senior centers in the city. Some of the wheelchair bound people are pushed to activities by their friends, and snatches of overhead conversation indicate shared interest and concerns. Neither group seems out of place. Yet, this is neither a nursing home nor your-run-of-the-mill center. It seems to have achieved an enviable balance.

The scene is the ARC Ft. Washington Senior Center, where two agencies, the center itself and Selfhelp Community Services, have reached the final stage of a long process of integrating the handicapped elderly into the program. How this happened, what made it work and the pitfalls along the way are the basis for this article. In particular, the widespread and differential use of groups—formal and informal—large and small, has been the modality of choice for doing the bulk of the work.

Harriette Friedlander, ACSW, is the Director of Social Services, Selfhelp Community Services, New York, New York.

The Author wishes to acknowledge the use of reports and other work submitted by Frances Adler, and Maria Brown on the first stage of the program and by Roberta Sackman on the later period.

© 1983 by The Haworth Press, Inc. All rights reserved.

The program, known as the Hillside Aged Program, was started in 1973 by Selfhelp Community Services in a converted kindergarten building in Washington Heights. Since Selfhelp's founding in 1936, when a group of refugees from Nazi persecution banded together to help other refugees, the agency's hallmark of service has been the new, the flexible, and the innovative.

During this time, the agency's social service staff was, and indeed still is systematically serving the bulk of their clients through home visiting. The client group is frail elderly who are being maintained in their homes through a variety of adequate and often not so inadequate arrangements.

Not yet in need of nursing home care, this group was truly isolated and alone. Some of them had not left their homes in many years, and the majority of their social contacts were through the visits of their social worker, perhaps a visiting nurse, and any family members that they may have had. Social contacts are further limited by the period of isolation that did not allow people to maintain their old contacts in the world, as well as the gradual dwindling of the neighborhood support systems in the Washington Heights area.

In its search to provide a service to these clients, the agency began to develop the concept of a small day center that would provide a home away from home for them. The program design was to provide a day center for those handicapped elderly who were able to be maintained in their homes, yet were isolated during the day. The aim of the program was to maintain the clients in the community for as long as possible by preventing institutionalization, to provide a place for socialization and interaction, to provide relief for family members who were caring for handicapped members in their homes, and to enable these isolated people to relate better to their families and caregivers by providing a laboratory for interactional skills.

Beginning discussions focused around the benefits of the medical model versus the social model. Then, as now, in-home services were focused on rehabilitation. Many disabled elderly, after reaching optimum functioning through rehabilitation services are either discharged from the hospitals or from their in-home nursing care. Large senior centers are big, noisy places where people have to fend for themselves, and any help for activities of daily living, such as dressing, toileting, or feeding, is not available. Door to door transportation was nonexistent. Even though the medical model had many benefits, including the concentration of services under one roof, and the potential for stable funding, the agency opted for the social model as truly filling a gap in service to this population. The first step, after rehabilitating the building and obtaining medical back up from the community hospitals, was to recruit potential members. For people who had been locked in to their homes for as many as seven or eight years, the prospect of going down to the street, much less to an unknown center, was terrifying. The agency began by selecting a small group of people who had been with the agency many years and who were receiving both home care and social services. Using the individual relationships with the caseworkers, a small planning committee was formed. The use of a small group was felt to be most manageable in terms of members comfort in reentering social situations. Five potential members met for a series of planning sessions to work out with the staff the possible program. In terms of the agency's planning, it was felt important to focus on the services most needed by this client group. In terms of the client population, there were a number of goals. First, there was a need to realistically ascertain how much responsibility this group could take for planning and implementing its own program. It was felt that by having the members take an active part in the preliminary planning they would be encouraged to develop and maintain important social roles. For this group, the customary, or expected losses of old age, in the areas of physical health, economics, vocational identification and loss of social roles had been magnified, and one of the most important goals was the restoration of self esteem by establishing new roles.

The members met with the social worker and the staff for a period of several weeks. Although this was ostensibly a task oriented group it allowed the members and the staff a mini laboratory to work out some of the kinks in the program. As members felt that what they had to say mattered, that they would in fact exercise some control over their own lives, they began to move from fear and suspicion to acceptance and even assertiveness. Group meetings were marked by real movement from reliance on the staff to a real sense of shared work. For many years afterwards, this group would consider itself part of the founders of the program, and an informal steering committee.

After much discussion, the basic necessary services were agreed upon. Transportation was one of the first, and most essential services. The program could be great, but if no one could come, it really did not matter. Social services, therepeutic recreation, nutrition, and assistance in the activities of daily living were finally decided upon. To be eligible for the program, people had to be over 50, handicapped, living in the Washington Heights area, capable of participating in a group program, capable of deriving benefits from the program, and be under medical supervision. Screenings were done through home visits by the social worker. An essential part of the application was a visit to the center, for people to see what it might involve and meet the other members. For the new, and often frightened applicant, this was often the single most motivating experience for participation. In fact, at the beginning there was the unexpected problem of trying to sell this new service to the potential members. The reason behind this soon became clear. The typical candidate had been shut away and forgotten for so long that the thought of reentering a social situation was overwhelming. It was often only during the initial visit that the person could relate to fellow members and take a tentative step towards reentering the world.

By March of 1974 there were 23 members, and referrals were coming fast and furious. A new problem had come up. The program was being seen as a last resort, a place where people were being referred when anything short of a nursing home had failed. Pressure was being put on the program to accept people that could not benefit from the program, either because they could not follow the few simple rules or could not tolerate a full days exertions. The primary problem was with the mentally frail. Although in the beginning there were idealistic hopes about integrating the mentally and physically frail, this soon proved impossible. Visions of the mentally frail assisting the handicapped with physical activity, and the handicapped guiding and monitoring the more mentally handicapped disappeared. It became obvious that each group had its own problems and at this stage had little left to give out. This was the first major crisis in the group as a whole. There was much discussion and debate among the members, the staff and the agency, and a decision was made to accommodate primarily the physically handicapped.

At this juncture, the group consisted of 29 members, 21 women and eight men. The age range was from 52 to 84, with an average age of 67.72% were being medically followed, the rest were not. 35% were in wheelchairs, 49% were ambulatory with the aid of a cane, 6% needed walkers, and the rest required no devices. 79% required ambulette transportation. 55% lived alone, and only 38% received SSI. As a group, there was a wide range of ethnic and racial integration. All members had more than one chronic disease. The primary disabilities, in rank order were strokes, legal blindness, multiple sclerosis, cardiac problems, osteoarthritis, rheumatoid arthritis, hip fractures, sight problems, depression, gastrointestinal problems, neurological disorders, spondylitis, bilateral hip dislocation, and amputation.

The program went through a number of changes, eventually reaching a membership of 55, with an average daily attendance of 25. A strong network of services among other agencies in the community developed, and clients received a wide range of support service. Scheduling people with serious ADL needs was worked out so that the nurses aide could provide maximum use of time. Through a grant of public funds, the program acquired its own busses. This enabled it to provide the additional services of transportation to medical and other appointments as well as group outings.

On a routine day at the center, the ambulatory members would begin to arrive about 9:30. The staff would use the early morning time to prepare for the day, take care of last minute scheduling changes, etc. The vans would start to deliver members shortly after 10 AM although there were often delays due to weather, illness and mechanical failure. During arrival time, coffee was served, newspapers were distributed and read, and it was a time of quiet discussion among members and staff. Once all the members were present, there was a general community meeting, open to all members and lead by the social worker. The topics covered were wide ranging, and included informational sessions, current events, and topics much more personal in nature. This aspect of the program was considered very important, and was the one activity in which every member participated. Levels of participation varied from just sitting and absorbing the feelings and communality of the group to actively participating. Although the center's policy was that no member be forced to attend any activity, when some members choose to avoid this meeting it became the topic of discussion for the whole group. The members finally decided that everyone should be present, and brought a good deal of peer pressure to bear on those who had chosen to absent themselves.

The range of topics covered gave the members a chance to practice a variety of interactions and social roles. Current events was often part of the agenda, and there was a strong emphasis placed on matters affecting the handicapped. This provided a non-threatening forum for beginning discussion of handicaps and how they affect daily living. Analysis of work with chronically ill patients shows how the shared experience and the accepting atmosphere of the group can encourage mutual support and discussion of the full impact of members conditions. As members began to trust, understand, and tolerate each other, they began to admit their vulnerabilities and share their anger, frustration, hopelessness and fears. They began to recognize their shared struggles, to help and accept one another and to share jointly in problem solving, both for the program and each other.

Another important aspect of this discussion was that it gave the newer, the more fearful, or the most reticent members a chance to be part of the group at a relatively low personal risk. For new members in particular, the act of just showing up made them part of the whole. They could observe the social roles taken by people with whom they could identify, and had a chance to evaluate for themselves how they might wish to begin to take more active roles.

The other benefit of this meeting was that it gave the members a chance to participate actively in decisions affecting the program. It was a chance to control something, to influence their lives in a way that had been all but abandoned by many of them. It gave them a chance to exercise autonomy and assertiveness in a relatively safe arena. This large group discussion went on until noon, when everyone went in for lunch. Although lunch had been planned for relaxed eating and socialization, it turned out to be much more focused on simply eating. It also provided a "cool-out" period for the members after the business of the morning. In the afternoon, a variety of programs were offered on a voluntary basis. The keynote was flexibility and voluntary participation. Programs ranged from fairly passive activities, such as watching a film or sitting in the garden, through individual craft activities and small group discussions. This was also a time when people could meet with the social worker, arrange medical appointments, or just visit. When planning any activities for this kind of group, the physical limitations imposed by the clients abilities must be kept in mind. For many of them, the ability to actively participate was often quite limited by their pressing physical problems. Group work with this population was essentially of three types, each encouraging different levels of participation, each with its own goals and each achieving different results.

## Large Group Services

These services are exe  ,..fied by the prior detailed description of the Morning Meeting. Goals of these sessions included the pa..: 'pation of members in the decisions making process, as well as facilitation of independent functioning by identification with the stronger more articulate members. It also provided a way for members to feel like part of a group even if they were afraid of relating on a more intimate level. Other large group services included relatively passive activities, such as movies or lectures, which allowed the more frail isolated to join in with others at a low level of risk and involvement. They could also stay on the periphery of the larger discussion group without pressure to actually participate. This served the function of enhancing their self esteem and giving them practice in relating to others. For the more active members, leadership positions in the large group served in some way as a replacement for lost social roles. For many of them it was the first time that they could focus on issues outside their physical disabilities or the minutia of family life, and use their dormant intellectual and interpersonal skills. The large group activities also encouraged a strong identification with the program and proved to be a major source of support during the many changes that the program later faced.

## Formal Small Groups

These groups were time limited groups formed by the social worker to deal with specific issues. The very first group, as previously mentioned, was the Steering Committee. A tape of "introductions" made by this group at the beginning clearly reflect their feelings of inferiority, loneliness, depression, and low self esteem. As this group worked together and were actively solicited for advice and input into the program design they emerged as leaders within the larger program. Their experience also allowed them to become the role models for the newer members over the years.

Other types of groups were discussion groups in various foreign languages, that used the language as a tie to share experiences in daily living. Groups met to discuss the problems of relating to family members, husband, children, or other caregivers. Members would share advice and offer suggestions for dealing with the tension, hopelessness, resignation, or anger frequently experienced by the caregivers in their lives.

## Informal Small Groups

Since members were in the center together over a period of time, this tended to be the most frequent and useful modality. It was difficult to get certain members to join a formal group meeting, it was much more acceptable for the women working on needlepoint and embroidery to work together while they discussed some of their problems and methods for solving them. The social work role in this group was very different from that in the more formal groups. Rather than present content and act as an initiator and mediator, the worker here used the participant observer approach. She would act as facilitator of group interaction. She would often share some of her own observations and concerns, thus allowing members the possibility of opening themselves up to the others. Groups were both regular, such as the sewing group or the mens card group, and transitory, such as those people who would find themselves together in the garden. There was a real effort on the part of the staff to draw even the most isolated members into the informal group structure. This network of groups served many functions for the members. It enabled some of them to form friendships that maintained themselves through telephone contact when they were at home. It provided an important forum to air their complaints and share coping strategies. They were able to provide each other with practical suggestions for managing at home and in the community. Together they were able to attempt things that they were afraid to do alone. This might include shopping trips or trips to the movies. For people who had, until this point, not left their apartments in years, a trip to the movies was a major event, to be anticipated actively, enjoyed to the fullest, and discussed and rediscussed for months afterwards. This network also served to welcome new members. A welcoming committee would adopt each new member and take responsibility for orienting them to the center. In terms of feeling more in control of their lives, members would actively participate in discussions with local community representatives that would come to the center. Members learned from each other how to be their own advocates in the area of entitlements and concrete problems, and would either do this from the center or discuss strategies at the center to be carried out at home. The strength and bonding that developed in the members would serve them in good stead during the crisis and changes that occurred in the program in the following years. Two years after the programs inception, Selfhelp was faced with the problem of shrinking private funds and the necessity of closing the center. Because HAP was based on a social rather than a medical model, repeated efforts had not been able to secure any government funds for the program and the agency could no longer support it on purely private donations. Although the members contributed a modest amount, it did not serve to cover the incredible cost of the program. The members did not sit idly by and watch their program be closed down. It had become more than just an escape for them—it had taken a group of people whose handicap had made them social outcasts and had offered them an opportunity to meet others, to communicate with others, and to share in the activities of the world. It had provided them with friends, coping mechanisms, and an outlet to the real world. They did not give up and return to their former imprisonment easily. They were able to use their new self esteem to focus efforts and attention at maintaining HAP. They met with Selfhelp administration and local officials. They wrote letters, they got on television and they turned it around. Muhammed Ali saw their show on television and came over to donate the funds to keep the center functioning for another year. It was a year, maybe not forever, but it was something the members had done themselves. It is hard to measure success, but when you look at a group of physically frail elderly who had seen themselves as invisible drains on society, it seemed hard to compare them with the group that sat cheering ''The Champ.''

In the year's time that the members' efforts bought, the agency was able to build a plan to continue the services of the program in a more manageable way. It was clear that the continued existence of the program was vital, it was also clear that there was no way Selfhelp or any other private agency could continue to pay for it alone, and that there would be no source of government money for a long time. Through incredible cooperation in the Washington Heights Community, plans were begun to move the center in with the ARC Ft. Washington Senior Center, one of the large Title 20 senior centers in the community. The transportation component, the nurses aide, social services, and the group recreation and discussion components were kept. The great, airy building, the garden, and the sense of specialness were lost. The members were able to accept the tradeoff, and the process of integration had begun.

Group support mechanisms had worked before, so an "Integration Group" was formed. A number of the more healthy members began to go to the ARC Center a few days a week to get the sense of the center and report back to the group what it was like. In truth, it was not the same as HAP—it was indeed one of the bustling foci of activities that had been too much for them at the beginning. But they talked about their choices—no one wanted to go back to sitting in their wheelchair staring at the window all day. They knew that there was more for them then that, so they decided they would just have to adapt. Coping skills that had begun to emerge in the protected atmosphere of HAP would have to be called on in stronger measure to get them through.

The agency plan was to work with the center to make it accessible to the handicapped of the community. The purpose of this was two fold. First, it would provide continuity of service for the HAP members. Second, it was felt that although the handicapped were not traditional users of the senior center, for reasons described earlier, that here the experience of the HAP program would enable this to become the first really integrated senior center in the city. There would be the additional benefit of enabling the frailer members of the senior center, those who had started out as healthy older adults but who were now frail themselves, to remain in the center where they had established ties. There was one final benefit—the center was founded by public money. This would enable to private funds to be used for those services that would go directly to the handicapped while enabling the handicapped to take advantage of the public funds to which they were entitled.

The integration of the handicapped and non-handicapped members was planned to occur in stages. This would allow both sets of participants to deal with the situation over a period of time. At first, the HAP members could only stay on the first floor of the center, although the main center of activities was in the basement below. It was planned for HAP to retain its separate identity for the first two years, with the eventual goal being integration into all the activities of the center. From the beginning, the staff of the Senior Center attempted to hold certain centerwide activities upstairs where the HAP members could participate. In addition, informal coffee was served in that location in the mornings so that people could begin to know each other.

As in the beginning of HAP, there has been a real emphasis on group activities. Large group activities, that allow for a variety of interactions have been helpful in allowing the members to feel each other out. Lectures, bingo, and arts and crafts have been particularly helpful in allowing the two groups to begin to know each other. The fear evoked in the healthier members, concerns about their own aging, resentments about the special services offered to the handicapped, fears of losing "their" center have all ameliorated as people in the two groups have begun to know each other. HAP members have made a real effort to participate in large group activities within their physical limitations. They have gone on large trips, and have asked to be carried downstairs to participate in festive events, such as Thanksgiving. In their now familiar small group forums they have begun to examine their concerns about the integration process and deal with their many losses. In the move, they did lose a lot of specialness, They also lost many of their familiar staff. What they did not lose during the integration was their membership. When the building closed, and people were transported to the new center, only one member did not make the transition. The meaningfulness of the program, and the commitment to maintaining themselves is apparent in their continued fight for active participation in their community.

In reviewing the experience, one sees its applicability to urban, suburban, and rural settings. Particularly in less densely populated settings, where there is little to see from your window that involves the hustle and bustle of daily living, the benefits of such a socialization program cannot be underestimated. The key services—transportation, assistance with activities of daily living, and widespread use of group support systems make the experience transferable and valuable. When one looks at the HAP participants today, it is hard to imagine they once were locked away in their apartments suffering from the extremes of social and emotional isolation that they had endured for so many years. They have reentered the world, and are using the new networks of support and encouragement to keep their place in it.

# THE GROUP:
# A CHANCE AT HUMAN CONNECTION
# FOR THE MENTALLY
# IMPAIRED OLDER PERSON

Judith A. Lee

ABSTRACT. This article describes an effective summer day program for the mentally impaired elderly. It discusses and illustrates the helping principles applied in a life model and interactionally oriented group and milieu approach. A sense of self is restored through community, and through providing opportunities for recall through community, and through providing opportunities for recall through doing, talking and sharing common feelings. The provision of a positive here and now experience which recognizes and bolsters strengths makes it more attractive to live more fully here and now. Even the most regressed patients improved in outlook and functioning as a result of the group experience.

> I grow older. . .I grow old. . .
> I shall wear white flannel trousers,
>     and walk upon the beach
> I have heard the mermaids singing,
>     each to each.
> I do not think that they will sing
>     to me.
>
> T.S. Eliot

## Introduction

The poet speaks of growing old with autonomy and dignity. Yet there is sadness in his feeling "they will not sing to me," that something symbolic of love, adventure and connection is, he thinks, now denied him. How much more is the depression and anxiety compounded when one begins to forget who one is, where one wants to go, how to get there, what to wear, where one has been, or momentarily who a loved one is. An "intact," older person may find value in interaction with others, or in memory. But we are

Judith A. Lee, DSW, is an Assistant Professor of Social Work, New York University, School of Social Work.

© 1983 by The Haworth Press, Inc. All rights reserved.

intolerant of those who "become senile," "regress," "forget," and otherwise show signs of "brain damage." The threat is too great, it could happen to us. Moreover, with all of our technology, we can not reverse or arrest genuine deteriorative processes. Paradoxically, we pull away our support as we angrily face the sheer frustration that there is no "Cure."

This article will describe a specific mutual aid group and milieu approach to this neglected population (Schwartz, 1971; Gitterman and Germain, 1980). The group described was the eleventh such group in a "Summer Day Camp Program" originally conceived and developed by social work administration and staff at a large general Hospital (Putter, 1967).[1] This author built upon the existing program and further conceptualized and developed some of the practice principles applied.[2] The unique approach of the program, and the practice implications will be discussed. The time period is the summer of 1976 although the program continues to date. The group met for seventeen days, twice a week throughout the summer. Patients were bussed to a recreation room with a kitchen and outside garden in a nearby Housing Complex. The patient staff ratio was one worker to six patients.[3] Although roles were defined, each staff person also took direct practice roles with the group members.

## The Population

The program was designed to serve mainly the more confused and disoriented patients who did not fit in other hospital or community programs. The sources of referral were from the Skilled Nursing Ward, the Geriatric Mental Health Service, the Home Care Department, and the general Outpatient Department. The program, a part of the Social Work Department offered services to all related areas of the Hospital. Twenty-six individuals were served and fifteen attended regularly. Fourteen more severely disoriented patients attended, six of whom were also paranoid. The twelve additional members were seriously depressed people, each with medical and social problems compounding their sense of loss.[4] For example, Mr. Stein, age

---

[1]The program was developed at The City Hospital Center at Elmhurst, Mt. Sinai Hospital Services, Elmhurst, New York. Helen Lokshin, Chief of Social Services and author of many articles on the ill elderly, conceived of and guided this program's development This author is indebted to her for guidance and inspiration in working with this population. Jerry Allford, Assistant Chief also provided consultation.

[2]Director of the Program in 1976, hired under a special grant.

[3]The Program was expertly staffed by Edythe Scharlop, MSW Senior Social Worker, overall director since 1967, Susan McGuiness, BSW, Social Worker, Genevieve Boyce, Nurse's Aide, and John Mintz MSW, Gerontology Fellow.

[4]See Ban (1978) for a connection between depression and organic brain syndrome.

94, was rapidly losing both sight and hearing. Mrs. Green just retired from her chambermaid's job at 82. Mrs. Charles, a gentle somewhat paranoid West Indian lady of 81, was depressed about living in a foster home. Although they were more "intact," several had begun to lie in bed all day at home, not care for their personal needs and have crying spells. The age range in the group was from 64–100 with most in their 80s. Several needed toileting and help in ambulation and eating.

## The Use of Activities

The best programming is related to the life experiences of the group members. Since most of our population had lost spontaneity, the group usually could not be asked to initiate suggestions. We worked at striking a balance between providing opportunities that would evoke recall, and rekindle former interests and skills—and being attentive listeners who could elevate recall into activities of interest to the group. The activities reflect the attempt at providing structure without over-structuring and building in the element of choice without raising anxieties over choosing. Ms. Lokshin felt choice was critical to the program. She notes that "In meeting health needs human needs were sometimes restricted." The autonomy represented in the act of choosing is critical to human beings.

Activities were related to the goals of providing opportunity for: The recall of former social skills and memories toward the restoration of the self-concept (Pincus, 1967); to move from isolation toward meaningful interaction and the forming of relationships (Germain, 1979); to gain acceptance and respect from others; for competence and mastery (Maluccio, 1979); and to simply find new enjoyments in life-enjoyments of doing, going, and being more comfortable with self and others.

One does not work on a self-concept by simply doing things with people or talking about who they were. The skill of the worker is to develop a fine sense of who the individual member is and to draw this out. It takes much time and skill to learn who elderly people are, particularly when they can only reveal themselves very indirectly, subtly and slowly. The discovery process with each member, therefore, was like a careful archaeological search for the precious artifacts representing the sense of self.

## Activities Related to Dressing and Appearance

For many the opportunity to get "dressed up" was a new one. The Nurse's Aide who helped dress the ward patients each day took special care to encourage choice and discussion. Soon they were speaking of wanting to wear undergarments, jewelry and make-up "to look more alluring." Mrs. Flynn, who lives alone at home, began the program wearing the same dress each time but eventually won acclaim from the group for the pretty dresses she wore. Out of this revitalized interest in dress and appearance, several activities emerged such as mending, making jewelry, and photography.

*A Polaroid camera* was used as a dimension of opening up a new experience that had immediate impact. Several commented "Is that me? I look a lot better than I thought." They also began to compliment each other and attempted to call each by name "look at Mrs. er-What's your name? How nice you look!" It also brought a discussion of age and time in its positive and negative aspects.

*A Slide show* and color prints taken at different points in the program was used in the same way, and to assist in review of the experience as part of the termination process. Each person received his or her own picture and a group picture and made an album to save them in.

*Portraiture.* Miss Donnelly, age 88, had been a professional artist. However, she had no art materials in her home and had not done art work in years. She was extremely forgetful and confused. Yet, when given crayons and stick water colors, she did lively portraits of other members of the group. The others valued them and made comments like "That's really me, I can see myself in that." Her esteem in the group soared. Overall a norm of trying to "look nice" emerged in the group and those who took extra care were noticed by the group. This encouraged attention to appearance and added to a positive sense of bodily self.

## Activities Related to Regaining Earlier Skills

*Negotiating stairs, riding the bus.* For several, unused motor skills had been forgotton. For Mrs. Vales, an alcoholic hospitalized for two months, the bus stairs brought bewilderment. The command to "go upstairs" brought a sitting down and reeling backwards. After negotiating stairs in the garden she did somewhat better on the bus stairs on the way home. To staff's surprise the next time she walked up the bus steps easily. Several also asked how much they needed to board the bus which brought discussion of fares, senior citizen's card and the high cost of living. The sights seen on the bus trip were highlighted by workers and discussion of members' neighborhoods ensued.

*Going to stores.* Volunteers accompanied the worker to the supermarket for something needed for lunch. This involved looking at the stores, becoming aware of available merchandise, prices, etc. This was most effective reality orientation as prices became real and they realized for example that homemakers were not cheating them. The dignity of choosing and making the purchase ws a new experience.

*Lunch Preparation.* Mrs. Tallon, a French woman, was moderately confused and paranoid. She was sometimes bitter, critical, and often aggressive toward other ward patients, but almost always friendly and smiling with the staff. By rediscovering her fine culinary skills she was able to contribute to the group and in turn, receive from them. Mrs. Flynn proudly recalled that she had been a waitress, and never missed an opportunity to be helpful. She began to have more confidence in her abilities to communicate as she had been well aware of her problems in forgetting words and thoughts mid stream. On one occasion when she served the bus driver she returned to the group beaming, saying "I spoke to him for quite a while and he *listened* to me!" She also identified with the less forgetful members who readily accepted her. Her motivation for attending the group was so high that once she wore her shoes to bed at night so she would be ready in the morning!

Group members had satisfaction in helping produce their own luncheon and a sense of self as a competent homemaker was restored for many. However, there was sensitivity to the fact that some had not been homemakers and felt more awkward than reassured. It was not expected that all members participate in the same way. Provision was made for many other areas of accomplishment in the program.

*Stimulation of memory and mastery through music and art.* Almost all members loved to sing old time songs and ethnic music. Records were played often. Mrs. Iskoti, a ward patient with Korsakov's syndrome was able to remember the words to many songs and her pride and joy in this was obvious. When Spanish music was on, Mrs. Santos who whined all day for her ills, was able to stop and enjoy, practically dancing in her seat. Mrs. Rothstein, a Home Care patient with severe forgetting, was particularly excited by a record called "Memories of Old Time Radio." She recalled soap operas and commercials. When there was tension in the group, such as paranoid accusations, members would suggest playing the records, which had a calming effect. Singing on the bus was another favorite.

Books of old time stage and screen stars were enjoyed and evoked further recall. Mrs. Fiore, a ward patient who functions on a confused infantile level, surprised everyone by accurately recalling accurate histories of her favorite stars. This helped others to react to her as more than the "one with no sense" as they usually labeled her, for at least a little while. Current newspapers were also enjoyed.

A variety of pictures were used as part of a decoupage project. As group members chose pictures each associated to its personal meaning: a church and religion; an American Eagle and the wars remembered, and so on. Mrs. Rothstein chose a caricature of a mouse couple getting married. For the first time she spoke of her own marriage and her long deceased husband. Her sense of loss was apparent and members sympathized fully with her. Mr. Stein, who can see very little, chose a picture for his grandson and glued it himself, feeling the edges of the plaque. His family was delighted with his "work" and he always asked to participate in the crafts. At times the group members also enjoyed pasting pre-cut forms on paper, as this demanded less skill and spontaneity. Several other simple but decorative projects were also accomplished. Members were happy with both the finished project and the feeling of mastery in doing it.

*Table Games* and throwing a ball while seated in a circle were also enjoyed. The table games had to be supervised or members generally forgot how to play. Playing ball was cause for laughter and joy.

*Outings*

A favorite part of the program was simply being out of doors at the State Park and in the garden at the Apartments. Outings were limited to spots accessible to the bathroom and good weather. As they got to know each other better and the group moved into a closer intimacy, the times outdoors seated in a circle enabled very relaxed, spontaneous interaction and discussion to appear. By the middle of the program, just being together in a relaxed way was beneficial.

On one occasion five ward patients went on a trip to a neighborhood diner. Each strove to meet the expectations of "eating out." Table manners were improved. There was a light, humorous and open mood. Mrs. Steiner was able to share very poignant feelings about embarrassment over her "forgetting." This small nonjudgemental homogeneous group seemed more tension-free than the larger group, perhaps enabling a different kind of work to emerge.

For the last outing, the group members decided to go to Jahns' Ice Cream Parlor. They saw it as a special treat which recaptured earlier days for them. The activities provided content in empty lives, opportunities for competence, mastery and enjoyment (Maluccio, 1981) and allowed for recall to emerge as they connected to parts of their lives now forgotten. Activities were not prescribed, but meaning was found in the range, choice, and intrinsic reward of activities. Reality was reinforced by living it, not merely by talking about it.

## Talking–the Content Themes

Structured talk times, and capitalizing on spontaneously emerging discussion were critical parts of the program. Yet we must bear in mind that we often measure the importance of words differently from the importance of doing, while all are part of the same process (Shulman, 1971).

### Beginnings

There was initial ambivalence around the new experience—looking forward to it but with fears of leaving the ward (or home), of being lost, of not knowing where they were going or why despite explanations. This was handled by the workers with patient explaining, verbal and non-verbal reassurances, and by helping other members to offer reassurances. Timidity and a natural reticence with others was handled by the workers with an invitation (often repeated in different ways) to tell a little about who they are, name, age, where from, former work, etc. As each was able to give a little and feel less self-conscious, the workers established commonalities between members—who came from Europe, or from New York, what occupations were similiar and so on. They were openly told the purposes of the group and their input was invited as it was available, thus forming a contract.

### Ongoing Working Themes

*Embarrassment and frustration at forgetting* words in mid-sentence was an important feeling theme which emerged early in the process. This was handled by recognizing the feelings and asking if others had experienced similar problems with forgetting.

*Appropriate Behavior.* The expression of feelings and worries around severe deviant behavior in the group, e.g. bizarreness, or paranoia, or patients who cry and moan that they "want to go home" all day were common. Norms developed around appropriate behavior, and members were helped by each other to live up to the norms.

*Reminiscences.* Who am I, Who was I? With the many efforts made to evoke recall and reminiscing much of the talk was around who they were in the past, jobs held, raising children, family of orientation, etc. Miss Donnelly, for example, who seemed to have forgotten all, suddenly remembered while sketching flowers in the garden that she had been a "canteen girl" during W.W.1. in France and that the flowers on the mountainside were similar to these. She was proud of her role in the war effort and enjoyed this new recall. This helped others to remember what it was like in the war years for them.

The workers constantly responded to the slightest cue that evoked memories, making connections from one person's memories to another (Pincus, 1967).

## The Here and Now

As many of the more confused patients had trouble with present orientation, a here and now approach was used. For example, when Mrs. Iskoti or Mrs. Fiore would speak of themselves as little girls "Daddy brought me these shoes, he'll get mad if I scuff them, " the workers gently let them know they were mature women whose parents had died a long time ago. Discussion followed of who was now in their family and where they were now. A goal was to make the here and now more attractive to live in.

A key contribution of the program was the working out of every day living problems. Older persons desperately need to gain some control over the systems they must negotiate (Miller and Solomon, 1979). For example, Mrs. Charles often discussed her unhappiness in her foster home. The workers helped clarify her desire to be cared for, and her fears of being left alone when the foster family was out. Alternatives to foster homes were discussed. The workers helped her rehearse with the group what she would like to say to her planning social worker around the kind of living situation she would like.

She and several others were also able to share their disappointments in the lack of attention paid to them by their children or family. Mrs. Flynn, for example, praised her daughters but bitterly told of her son sending her a card once a year. Workers related to the member's anger and disappointment directly and gently.

Several patients who lived alone at home expressed how difficult this was. Workers helped them tell how they managed in order to help each other with suggestions. Workers also helped them explore their needs for more Home Attendant services. Miss Donnelly for example, who had been too proud to accept all but a few hours a day was able to acknowledge her need for someone on a 24-hour basis, saying "Now that I've been with people all day, I don't want to stay alone." This was very important as her severe forgetting was dangerous, a pot was seen burning on the stove and she was totally unaware of it.

As others discussed their difficulties in daily management we arranged team conferences with their workers to explore alternatives. And, in team conference we explored whether several were certified as legally blind and eligible for services to the blind.

## Illness and Other Losses

Loss of spouses, children, friends, family, health, status, functioning and memory were frequent topics of discussion. The worker's role in this was to help them share and find comfort in a common situtation, to express the pain, but not "hit them over the head" with it. For example, on one occasion while sitting in the garden Mrs. Rothstein spoke of the loss of her sister while they were both adolescents. The group was sympathetic and Mrs. Charles spoke of the loss of her sister a few years ago. Mrs. Fiore walked away and started crying. The worker reached out. She said "she didn't want to talk about it" but rejoined the group. She then told of losing her daughter to a fatal illness at age 18. There was empathy from all, then a silence. The worker commented on the hard times they've all had. Members' comments were to the effect that these things happen to all of us in life. One group member then began to talk of enjoying the garden. The worker commented that that was enough of the sad memories for today, huh? They laughed and changed the theme easily.

The loss of present functioning on a physical and mental level was another key theme. Everyone would comment at various points of "How I used to be," of "How I could do that only a few years ago." The members themselves could also give themselves credit "Look at me at 94, I'm still going strong," which was supported and encouraged. An underlying theme was illness, coping with the sickness itself, and with doctors, diets, and operations. Yet considering all were ill and under the doctor's care, it was surprising that this was not a more dominant preoccupation.

## Where Am I Going?

This was perhaps the most difficult area and one in which both workers and members used some avoidance. It was easy to focus on moving from the ward to a Health Related Facility or home with a homemaker. For example, a worker helped Mrs. Tallon to express her feelings about being discharged from the ward on one day's notice. She expressed her fears of leaving the routine of the hospital and her friends in the hospital and day camp. When she was assured that she could still come to the day camp she was delighted, "Oh, it is all right then, I will not lose my friends." But fears of fatal illness or death were raised in disguised way ("Don't trust the doctors,'' or "I'm afraid to be alone" or "sit near me and hold my hand, I don't feel well"). Those who were more intact could talk of death easily and had become philosophical in a positive way. While the others heard this and agreed, deeper fears were generally not explored except on a one-to-one basis. Staff was simply unsure of how much the more confused members could handle in the group. The group climate, with several people often talking at one time did not often lend itself to this.

An example of handling these feelings in the one-to-one follows. Mrs. Terillo, age 94, was an emotionally demanding woman who clutched on to workers as on to life. As response was given throughout the summer, she was able to share with a worker that recently "she dreamed that her husband (long deceased) came and told her he was waiting for her." Former dreams had him turning his back and going away. You were frightened the worker said. Yes, I think he was inviting me. Pause. You mean dying, the worker asked. Yes, she replied, but I'm not ready to go. I worry about things . . . The worker asked what she worried about, and continued to stay with Mrs. Terillo on this most difficult theme. It is significant that members knew dying was not a taboo subject in this group.

*Termination and Transition Themes—The Meaning of the Day Camp Experience*

As summer moved toward an end, the members shared feelings of missing the Day Camp. This was a place to go, to make friends, to be with people, why does it have to end? No matter how explicitly facilities in the community were discussed, most of our members would not be able to follow up. Staff had to help them express feelings about the loss of this vital link to people without offering false promises. For individuals we were able to make some connections. But mostly the work was to help them own the positive gains they had made this summer and say goodbye, encouraging those who were able to keep contact with each other by telephone. Workers and members alike joined in their wish for an ongoing Day Program throughout the year.

## The Group Process And Special Dynamics

The group was a large and heterogeneous gathering of people who had the common bond of advanced age, illnesses of various sorts, including organic impairment, and difficulty in functioning. The abilities, damage, differences, and strengths among patients was striking and at times apparently too divergent. The examples given throughout this account indicate that mutual aid did indeed take place, and acceptance and understanding were available healing factors. But, some of the overall group dynamics were problematic. For example, there was an "ingroup" and "outgroup" with Mrs. Iskoti and Mrs. Fiore described by the others quite openly at times, as "having no marbles" or "no sense at all." This happened when they were particularly regressed or paranoid. These kinds of tension were difficult for the group to tolerate and made for negative experiences. In determining group composition, a gauge may be to weight the degree of deviance a member may have from the norm in the group. Some deviation is probably good. Vast deviation in either direction may mean problems. The staff and group members agreed that the best days were when attendance was about 12–13 and when no one group member demanded all staff time. The possibility of working with small sub groups independently within the program can also be considered.

The systematic ripple effects of being in the group also had a salutory effect on both patient and staff. For example, the heightened interest of nursing staff in the ward patients who participated, or in the Home Attendant/and/or Family becoming more involved in order to help prepare patients for the program twice a week. Also staff was better able to assess functioning and needs of the patients. They felt more rewarded in their own efforts. Therefore, several ward discharges were made and Home Attendant service was increased and so on. It is difficult to isolate any one factor as most helpful. Instead we look at individual progress as a response to the total impact of the program.

In terms of staffing the program, the team effort and decision-making input is effective, with the Director having final decision-making power. Staff often "pulled together" in a unique and beautiful way. It was also helpful for staff to share their own emotional responses in a mutual aid sub-group where one could laugh, cry, strategize and share knowledge and experiences in support of each other and the program. While there was never total agreement each of us learned much from the views of the others. The most critical question is around the continuation of the program throughout the year. The Program serves a population not served. Most group members move back to nothing at the close of the program. It is better to serve partially (over the summer) than not at all. But it is best to serve according to client need. These are clients who need this service on a year-round basis. A Day Hospital Program would fill the service gap (Bradshaw et al., 1980).

## Conclusions

A sense of self is restored through community, through providing opportunities for recall through doing together with some assurance of success, and the opportunity to talk, share feelings and help each other. The provision of a positive here and now experience which recognizes and bolsters strengths and self-confidence, makes it more attractive to live more fully in the here and now. Even the most regressed and deteriorated of the patients improved in outlook and functioning as a result of the group experience. The methods used are the three-fold approach of stimulating mutual aid and group process, and using doing and talking as vehicles of communication. Doing and producing restores a sense of self as a competent person. Talking and expressing feelings restores a sense of self as an intelligent person whose feelings are important to others. Some level of problems can also be "worked out" verbally. A sense of self is found in communication with others. The ability to form relationships, happily, supercedes the inability to conceptualize them. The sense of fellowship with peers and younger persons and the family-like primary group properties of the group, make for the necessary sense of belonging, respect, understanding and acceptance to those who have lost most primary group ties. In addition to Day Programs, this approach can be used on skilled nursing wards, geriatric wards, Health Related Facilities and Nursing Homes. There are some questions around optimum group composition to make the program even more effective. But, it must be overwhelmingly concluded that this population has strengths in making relationships and mutual aid which are usually underestimated. And, this group/milieu approach is a most effective way to serve the mentally impaired elderly.

## REFERENCES

Ban, T. "Aspects and Treatment of Organic Brain Syndrome." *Journal of Geriatric Psychiatry*, 11, 1978, pp. 143–148.

Bradshaw, B. R., Brandenburg, C., Basham, J. and Ferguson, E. "Long Term Care." *Journal of Gerontological Social Work*, Vol. 2 (3), Spring, 1980, pp. 185–198.

Euster, G. "Group Work Revisited: Directions for the Third Century." Social Work With Groups, Vol. 1 (2) Summer, 1978, pp. 207–214.

Germain, C. B., *Social Work Practice: People and Environments: An Ecological Perspective.* New York: Columbia University Press, 1979, p. 75.

Germain, C. B., and Gitterman, A., *The Life of Social Work Practice.* New York: Columbia University Press, 1980.

Maluccio, Anthony. *Promoting Competence in Clients: An Old/New Approach to Social Work Practice*, New York: The Free Press, 1981.

Miller, I. & Solomon, R. *The Development of Group Services for the Elderly: An Ecological Perspective.* New York: Columbia University Press, 1979, pp. 76–105.

Pincus, A. "Reminiscence in Aging and Its Implications for Social Work." *Social Work*, 12, July, 1967, pp. 33–41.

Putter, Zetta H. *Group Approaches in the Care of the Chronically Ill.* Journal of Jewish Communal Service, Vol. XLIV, No. 2, Winter 1967.

Schwartz, W. & Zalba S. *The Practice of Group Work.* New York: Columbia University Press, 1971.

Shulman, L. "Program in Group Work: Another Look." in Schwartz, W. and, Zalba, S. *The Practice of Group Work*. New York: Columbia University Press, 1971, pp. 221–240.

Weisman, C. B., *The Future is Now: A Manual for Adult Programs in Jewish Communal Service Agencies*, New York: National Jewish Welfare Board and the Brookdale Foundation, 1976.

# GROUP WORK WITH DISORIENTED NURSING HOME RESIDENTS

## Naomi Feil

ABSTRACT. This article presents the goals, rationale, history, and some implementing techniques to help disoriented old-old restore dignity and self worth in a group. The techniques focus on non-verbal helping methods. Validation/Fantasy is based on the following principles: 1) There is reason behind all behavior. 2) Each stage of life has different goals. 3) Goals of severely disoriented aged are to resolve the past. 4) Each human is valuable and unique. 5) The helper must use empathy and genuine human regard, tuning into the goals of the "other." 6) Damage to sensory cells can lead to a gradual blurring of present reality and self-awareness. 7) Early-learned emotional memory replaces cognitive thinking in disoriented aged. 8) Disoriented aged can tap logical thinking centers when they are helped to resolve the past. 9) Validation/Fantasy tunes into the old-old. Some prefer to remain in the past. Some can return to the present. No one formula works for everyone. 10) People who are disoriented and old-old and who cannot return to the outside community deserve to resolve the past and justify their past roles before death.

In 1963 I began Group Work with disoriented old-old residents at Montefiore Home for the Aged in Cleveland. The rational for group work with this population began in 1947 when Dr. Julius Weil, administrator of Montefiore Home, began his research. He found that the condition of the brain does not always relate to the behavior of old-old people in nursing homes. (Weil, 1966)[1] Autopsies showed that some residents with severe brain damage (Alzheimer's Plaques and neurofibrillary degeneration) functioned well until the moment of death. Other residents with little brain damage on autopsy were very disoriented. Dr. Weil's findings concur with pathologists reports investigating the aging process.[2] Dr. Weil found that group activities help re-motivate disoriented old-old residents,[3] providing, the worker used a nurturing approach.

My Social Group Work Goals were: to stimulate interaction; to establish roles; to motivate each individual towards renewed feelings of self-worth and usefulness in a Home for the Aged.[4] My therapeutic skills were actual-

Naomi Feil, ACSW, is the Consultant in Gerontology, Trainer and Group Worker, Amasa Stone Home VA Hospitals.

© 1983 by The Haworth Press, Inc. All rights reserved.

ly social group work techniques. I initially struggled to renew members' feelings of self worth through encouraging participation in the nursing home community and through orienting the disoriented residents to the reality of institutional living. I incorporated the Remotivation Techniques established in 1957 by Dorothy Smith in the Philadelphia State Hospital.[5] Utilizing some basic social work principles (e.g., meet the client where he/she is; each individual must *choose* to change; change evolves through a respectful, empathic, genuine, relationship with a helping person to meet the *client's* goals) I began by establishing a meaningful relationship with each prospective group member. Group members were "selected jointly by the psychiatrist, social workers and nursing staff..."[6] Criteria for group membership were: withdrawal from group participation or from interpersonal relationships and some capacity for verbalization. All members were selected from the Special Service Department for disoriented residents. (Special Service Department residents were those diagnosed as Senile Psychotic, Senile Demented, Ambulatory Schizophrenic, Chronic Organic Brain Damage, Arteriosclerotic with Organic Brain Syndrome, or Alzheimer's Disease." These labels changed from 1963 to 1981 with the diagnostic nomenclature prescribed by the American Psychiatric Association.[7])

After five years, I found that mixing mildly disoriented residents with severely confused residents was not helpful.[8] The more oriented residents did respond to Remotivation Technique Step 5: A Bridge to Reality—Reality Orientation. The more oriented residents were able to relate to objective program material. However, the disoriented residents who showed severe time confusion, could not and would not respond to reality orientation or objective program media. At the same time the more oriented residents were threatened and became hostile when facing severely disoriented peers in the group. By 1966, I found the goal of helping severely disoriented old-old people face reality to be unrealistic. Therefore, I abandoned this goal for severely disoriented residents when I found that these group members would withdraw, vegetate or become increasingly hostile whenever I tried to orient them to an intolerable reality.

I found that each such person was trapped in a world of fantasy.[9] Exploring feelings and reminiscing stimulated these group members to respond. Music stimulated their group cohesion and feelings of well being.

One severely disoriented old-old woman told me:

> Mrs. J: "It's better when you're crazy.
> Then, it doesn't matter what you do."

She explained this to me while singing, "Daisy, Daisy, I'm half crazy. . . ."
A second disoriented woman rose to leave the room:

>   Mrs. K: "I have to go home now to feed my kids."

>   N. Feil: "Mrs. K., you can't go home. Your children are not here.
>   You now live in a Home for older people-The Montefiore
>   Home."

>   Mrs. K: "I know that. Don't be stupid. That's why I have to leave.
>   Right now. I have to go to my OWN HOME TO FEED MY
>   KIDS."

No amount of presentation of reality could convince Mrs. K. She felt useless
in THE HOME. She wanted her own home. She wanted her own role as
mother of three children. She wanted to feel useful. *She wanted to be wanted
by someone she loved.* She withdrew from me, muttering:

>   Mrs. K: (pointing to me) "What does she know. Who does she think
>   she is?"[10]

Mr. Smith accused the administrator of castrating him in the attic. I tried
to reality orient Mr. Smith for three years. When the administrator retired,
Mr. Smith said to me:

>   Mr. S:   You're right. He didn't hurt me. I'm no good. I never was."

Those were the last words he spoke to me. He dropped his cane and never
walked again. On the rod of his wheelchair, he walked with his fingers, muttering the name of the street where he practiced law. He pounded his hurt
knee, muttering: "DAMN JUDGE, DAMN JUDGE. . . ." His sister told me
he never accomplished much. He blamed the judge, the administrator, the
doctor, God—all authority figures—for his own failures. His father had told
him: "You'll never amount to anything." Mr. Smith was castrated first,
through words, by his father. He had bottled up his rage, his hurt, his shame.
Now, in old-old age, his fury spilled to the surface. I refused to listen. I tried
to cork up his feelings by repeatedly telling him no one was hurting him.
He felt invalidated. He needed another human being to listen to him; to
validate him; to acknowledge that his *feelings*—(not his facts)- were true.[11]

Invalidated, he moved from 1) mild disorientation to 2) confusion in time
to 3) perpetual, repetitive agitated motion to 4) vegetation. Then he died.
Mr. Smith and hundreds of hundreds like him taught me to abandon reality
orientation with severely disoriented old-old people.

I separated the mildly confused who responded to reality orientation from the severely disoriented. The following criteria evolved through the years. These definitions helped select residents for groups that were appropriate for their needs.

*Stage One:*[1] *Occasional Disorientation*

- holds onto present reality
- can dress, toilet and control self
- can play games with rules
- has sense of humor
- wants to be reminded of present time and place
- has some sensory acuity and mobility
- resists change
- resents invasion of privacy
- denies strong feelings
- responds to current events groups, discussion groups and special interest groups

*Stage Two:*

A slow, progressive unfolding of feelings marks the retreat inward from occasional disorientation to severe disorientation. Adult controls fade. Sexual feelings emerge. Speech, social controls, awareness of clock time and reason slowly wane. Memory is selective and purposeful. People choose to remember pleasant material and forget painful facts.

*Stage 2: Time Confusion*

- Less communication with dictionary-words words now have personal, unique meanings (Example: *"Symofile,"* means similar, file, Feil. A former file-clerk says things are similar in Feil's group, by combining phrases.)
- Tenses change. People move back and forth in feeling time, not clock-time. Time is measured by one's life-time.[13]
- Open expression of feelings. Use of movements and rhythm replaces words.
- Vivid eidetic images replace visual acuity.
- Loss of sense of humor.
- Cannot obey rules when playing games.
- Forgets names, faces, places in present time.
- Remembers people and places with emotional meanings from the past.
- Responds to nurturing.

## *Stage 3: Repetitive Motion*

Disoriented residents who do not share feelings in Stage 2, move further inward. They retreat to early pre-language movements and sounds to nurture themselves. They return to the womb. They move to resolve the past, using their own body parts to represent people from the past.

- Repetitive sounds, clucking noises and rhythms
- Loss of self-awareness in time and space
- Loss of speech
- Increasing use of Symbols
- Responds to Nurturing

Residents in Stage One, *Occasional Confusion*, responded well in groups that required reality orientation. Residents in Stage Two and Three responded well in groups that validated their needs and their unique life goals. These validation groups acknowledged feelings. The worker uses empathy.

Empathy—walking in the shoes of the disoriented old-old person built trust. Trust brought security. Security built strength.

Strength brought feelings of self-worth. Self-worth reduced stress.[14] The worker's empathy revealed the following characteristics in disoriented old-old who were helped by Validation Groups:

Disoriented old-old return to the past to:
- Resolve unfinished business by expressing feelings that were hidden when controls were intact.
- Re-live past pleasures, replacing damaged intellectual thinking with feeling.
- Re-stimulate memories that provide continuity with useful roles.
- Re-treat from painful reality; from feelings of uselessness through Fantasy. (A perception of the world without using the sense organs.)

The worker can find empathy with the adolescent who slams doors, expresses raw emotions, and often acts "inappropriately." The middle-aged worker has been there. The worker has not been to the land of old-old age. Empathy is more difficult with disoriented old-old people—and gaining empathy—takes more time. Life-Goals in old-old age are quite different from middle-aged-adult-life goals. The old-old person returns to the past to resolve old conflicts, to justify living and prepare for dying. The old-old person who is disoriented in a nursing home, with *no hope of returning to the outside community* no longer wants to communicate with people in present time. They want loved ones from the past. They are not mindless. They are not demented. They survive the bleak present by holding onto past pleasures and resolving past conflicts. The worker with empathy understands the need to put aside middle-age, adult expectations. "Reason, think, control emotions, keep track of time, produce, communicate, use your head."

The empathetic worker tunes into the disoriented old-old person "where the client is." The worker understands *their* life-goals. The worker moves in tune to their life-rhythms, exploring their feelings, their acting-out behavior in order to build trust. The worker recognizes that each person is unique. There is no one formula for everyone. A trusting, nurturing relationship helps disoriented old-old people feel happier. The worker is *non-judgmental*, expecting progress according to the physical and emotional abilities of the disoriented old-old person.

When feelings are acknowledged they often diminish[15], become resolved and the person *chooses* to relate to present time and place. Disoriented old-old people respond best to Validation in a group. Genuine eye-contact, caring, touch, acknowledgment of usefullness in a group stimulates heightened interaction. Speech improves. Some become motivated to control "negative"[16] emotions. *Further deterioration lessens.* Never do physical, social and emotional factors combine to determine functioning as in old-old age.[17] When motivated, many disoriented old-old people tap dormant, logical thinking capacities and return to present reality -if they they feel nurtured and validated.

Our 1973 study showed that change in behavior is slow and fluctuates from day to day but permanent change does occur; that after 6 months of validation group meetings people diagnosed "organic brain damage" became less incontinent; speech improved; less crying, hitting, pounding, more smiling, talking, helping others; more awareness of external reality; more interaction outside of group meetings; greater contentment.[18]

The 1973 Study showed also: 2) that denial is the common life-time defense against stress. Disoriented old-old choose—on some level of awareness—to forget people and places that have little emotional meaning or satisfaction. They choose to remember people and places that will give strong emotional feelings of safety.[19] The old-old person who feels suddenly frail; who has avoided facing unpleasant issues in youth and middle-age; who now faces massive losses in old-old age must retreat. The life-long pattern of denial produces inflexibile coping methods. The person without the inner strength to defend himself against physical and social losses returns to the past for strength -in order to survive. They enter the Resolution vs.

Vegetation stage of living. They struggle to resolve the past to avoid vegetating until death. They now make closure with living. They now justify their existence by returning to the past. Carl Jung, Wilder Penfield, Eliot Slater, Piaget, Donald Hebb, Robert Ornstein[20] describe the early emotional thinking that precedes later-learning cognitive rational thought. Viktor Frankl adds:... "the prisoner finds a refuge from the emptiness and desolation...by escape into the past."[21]

Too many losses too late in life are too much to change a lifetime pattern of coping. The person has no choice but to retreat. When rational thinking centers become damaged, this ... "frees...and allows for greater non-verbal expression."[22] Early, emotional memories and fantasies replace later-learned logical thinking.

The group worker working with Disoriented Old-Old in Stage Two and Three understands their panic when facing an intolerable reality; their helpless frustration; their feelings of uselessness; their fear in being alone, abandoned by loved ones. The worker enters their inner reality and becomes a trusted significant other to decrease stress and increase self-worth.

The Validation Group produces energy. Stage Two and Three disoriented gain heightened awareness of themselves and others. They begin to risk interacting with each other as well as with the worker. They share universal feelings; Love, hate, fear of separation, struggles for identity and belonging. The worker's role is to find the universal feeling; share the feeling with group members; stimulate group members to help each other; gain group cohesion and feelings of well-being.

To form a Validation Group with Stage Two, Time Confused and Stage Three, Perpetual Repetitive Motion the following process was suggested:

1. Assess the stage of disorientation.[23]
2. Using questions that explore the past[24], take the history and establish trust in a one-to-one relationship.
3. Select 5–10 residents in Stage 2 and 3, (residents in Stage 1 benefit from reality-groups.)
4. Find a role for each group member. (Sample roles found in Implementing Manual.)[25]
5. Select: music, movement, topic, refreshments. (Sample of each in Implementing Manual.)
6. Involving the interdisciplinary staff in goal-setting for individuals and for the group; selecting a room with privacy; time and place for the meeting.
7. Arrange chairs in a small circle. Do not use a table. People need to sit close to hear and see and feel each other.

8. Follow the same ritual for the meeting each week. 1) welcome, 2) music, 3) discussion, 4) movement, 5) closing with refreshments.

Validation Group wrote these criteria for a worker when I was preparing to leave. All members were in Stage Two and Three Disorientation.

## SPECIAL SERVICE RESIDENT'S CRITERIA FOR GERIATRIC AID

1. A nice, gentle woman we can all get along with.
2. She must have a clear and low voice.
3. She must stay with us at least one year.
4. She should listen and talk and help people.

## FOOTNOTES AND BIBLIOGRAPHY

1. Weil, Julius, PhD "Special Program for the Senile in a Home for the Aged," *Geriatrics* 21 (Jan. 1966): 197–202.

2. Aker, J. B., Walsh, Arthur C., and Beam, J. R. *Mental Capacity Mental and Legal Aspects of the Aging.* New York: McGraw Hill Book Co., 1977.

3. Weil, Julius. "Pertinent Factors in the Development of a Special Service Department for the Senile in a Home for the Aged," *Fourth Congress of International Association of Gerontology.* Merano, Italy, July 14–19, 1957.

4. Feil, Naomi. "Group Therapy in a Home for the Aged," *The Gerontologist*, 7(3), Part 1 (September 1967).

5. Young, Clifford, Remotivation Coordinator, Research and Education Building, Philadelphia State Hospital, 14000 Roosevelt Boulevard, Philadelphia, Pennsylvania 19114.

6. Feil, Naomi. "A New Approach to Group Therapy With Senile Psychotic Aged," Unpublished paper presented at the 25th Annual Meeting of the Gerontological Society in San Juan, Puerto Rico, December, 1972.

7. The American Psychiatric Association, *Diagnostic and Statistical Manual*, I, II, and III. 1700 18th Street, N.W. Washington, D.C. 20009.

8. Feil, Naomi, "A New Approach to Group Therapy."

9. Ibid.

10. Ibid.

11. Feil, Naomi. *VALIDATION/FANTASY THERAPY*, New Manual Tells How to help Disoriented Old-Old, Edward Feil Productions, 4614 Prospect Avenue, Cleveland, Ohio 44103, 1981.

12. Ibid.

13. Feil, Edward Feil Productions, *100 YEARS TO LIVE*, Cleveland 1981, (16mm. Color-Sound Film.) 4614 Prospect Avenue, Cleveland, Ohio 44103, Dorsey-Paolini Scene.

14. Feil, Edward Feil Productions, *LOOKING FOR YESTERDAY* (Mrs. Kessler Scene,) Ibid. 16mm. Film.

15. von Franz-Hillman. *Jung's Typology.* Zurich: Spring Publications 1971.

16. Feil, Naomi. "Group Therapy in a Home for the Aged," *Ibid.* and "A New Approach to Group Therapy with Senile Psychotic Aged," Ibid.

17. Verwoerdt, Adrian, M. C. *Clinical Geropsychiatry*, Baltimore, Md.: The Williams & Wilkins Co., 1976.

18. Feil, Naomi, ''A New Approach to Group Therapy with Senile Psychotic Aged,'' Op. Cit.

19. Feil, Edward, *LOOKING FOR YESTERDAY, FILM CLIP, MRS. WARD.* (16 mm. Film, Edward Feil Productions, Producer.) 1980.

20. Ornstein, Robert E. *The Psychology of Consciousness.* New York: Harcourt, Brace Jovanovich, Inc., 1977.

21. Frankl, Viktor. *Man's Search for Meaning.* New York: Washington Square Press, 1963.

22. Zeidel. *Cerebral Correlations of Conscious Experience*; and Watzlawick, Paul. *The Language of Change.* New York: Basic Books, 1978.

23. Feil, Naomi, *VALIDATION/FANTASY THERAPY*, Op. Cit. page 22-33.

24. Feil, Naomi. *Validation/Fantasy Therapy.* Ibid. Page 36-37.

25. Feil, Naomi. *Validation/Fantasy Therapy.* Ibid. Page. 50-62.

Call for Papers

*Social Work with Groups* announces two forthcoming special issues
for which papers will now be received.

## GENDER AS AN ISSUE IN GROUP WORK

Guest Editors:  Dr. Charles Garvin
Dr. Beth Reed

School of Social Work
University of Michigan
1065 Frieze Building
Ann Arbor, Michigan 48104

DEADLINE:  December 15, 1982

## ETHNICITY AND GROUP WORK

Guest Editor:  Larry E. Davis, Assistant Professor

George Warren Brown School of Social Work
Washington University
Campus Box 116
St. Louis, Missouri 63130

DEADLINE:  January 15, 1983

Manuscripts should be sent to the guest editors.

# AN ADMISSIONS GROUP
# IN A SKILLED NURSING FACILITY

Sidney R. Saul

ABSTRACT. This paper describes the use of a group to help the frail elderly person during and immediately following admission to a skilled nursing facility. Within the framework of the interdisciplinary team, the group leader uses the group as a means of helping the new resident cope with the difficult change in living arrangements and concurrent circumstances posed by the need for total, skilled nursing care. The author offers a taped, verbatim record and shows how such a group serves both diagnostic and treatment purposes.

The new patient/resident in a skilled nursing facility usually arrives after having endured a series of traumatic life/health experiences. The older person is physically, psychologically and emotionally exhausted; may be dazed, confused, disoriented, angry—and is usually depressed and anxious. Having been subjected to a number of life threatening experiences, the person has for some time prior to admission, felt a loss of control over his or her own destiny.

In the Kingsbridge Heights Nursing Home, a 200 bed skilled nursing facility in the Bronx, NY the resources of the entire facility are mobilized to receive the newly admitted patient and to organize a coordinated, interdisciplinary care plan to 1) ease the trauma of admission and 2) develop treatment perspectives and methods. The Admissions group is one of these resources whose potential usefulness to a new patient is individually assessed and applied.

This group, therefore, is a mediating structure within the facility and may serve several purposes.

1. It is one way to help the new resident accommodate to this new, alien and very different living arrangement. The group affords an opportunity for socialization; for sharing and imparting important information about the setting and its various programs of care and service; for offering support—

Sidney R. Saul, EdD, CSW, is Coordinator, Psycho-Geriatric Services. Maimonides Community Mental Health Center, and Mental Health Consultant, Kingsbridge Heights Nursing Home, Bronx, New York.

© 1983 by The Haworth Press, Inc. All rights reserved.

both from peers and leader; and for providing a safe opportunity for ventilating feelings (which usually include anger, bewilderment and confusion as well as depression.)

2. This group also serves a diagnostic and treatment purpose, as it is one of several ways through which the staff may assess the social and intellectual capacities of the newcomer.

The use of memory exercises, stimulating intellect, challenging people to perform at their highest possible level of functioning, appealing to their mental and social health, using the group for mutual support—these are the treatment aspects. At the same time, the leader is assessing responses, checking reality contacts, observing the individual's capacity for relationship and communication; these are the diagnostic aspects of the group's contribution to the care plan.

## Referral to Group: Criteria and Process

Within a week after admission, the interdisciplinary patient care team meets to develop the plan of care for each new arrival. Reports from physician, nurse, social worker, dietician, activity and rehabilitation departments (OT and PT) are appropriately shared and a detailed plan is written re goals, expectations and interventions. This may include referral to the admissions group. Although there are no "hard-and-fast" rules regarding referral, some general criteria are applied to guide the team.

The resident who is clearly functioning on a high social and intellectual level—will be referred on to a number of appropriate groups and activities in the home: not necessarily to this group.

The resident who is too severely physically ill will *not* be considered for an admissions group.

The patient who shows extreme intellectual impairment; who at this point communicates only by shouting, moaning or other unintelligible sounds—will not be considered (note, however; such a person may be reassessed shortly afterward and referred, if appropriate).

The patient who presents a question as to social or intellectual adequacy and who can communicate—in any way—*is usually referred*. (In a 200 bed facility, this criteria offers sufficient candidates to hold such a group all year round).

The team's referrals are coordinated through the Social Service Department. The group leader reads the patient's chart to gather all relevant information and to review the interdisciplinary patient care plan (with attention to medications and drugs, as well as other specific treatment). There may be further discussion with, and clarification by, staff members (nurse, physician, activity, social service, rehabilitation, etc.) as may be needed.

The group leader then meets with the patient; checks the person's ability to communicate; discusses the nature and explains the purposes of the group and extends an invitation to attend. (The patient's consent is mandatory: no one is coerced. However, support from other staff members in encouraging attendance may be helpful. The newcomer may require reassurance from caring staff, such as the nurse's aide, etc. that attendance at the group will prove helpful to the patient. This suggests that all staff should understand the contribution of this group to patient care.)

The group is open-ended. Members may move in and out freely, as needed. Decisions to leave the group may be made by the patient; or recommended by the group and/or the leader.

## *The Group Session*

The following transcript presents a typical early session (the third) of such an admissions group. Participants have been admitted to the SNF within the past 3 months. The group has been assembled with the aid of the floor nurses.

### *Members*

Depressed: Mrs. Freed: Age: 85

Prior to admission, a mentally high functioning woman who had been a worker with handicapped people in a large agency. She had fractured her hip and suffered cardiac heart failure. She is currently wheelchair bound. Some memory loss noted by the team.

Depressed: Mrs. Tapok: Age: 84

Had worked as a housekeeper: suffered cardiac heart failure. Currently, exhibits general physical weakness and evidences some recent memory loss.

Depressed/Angry: Mr. Goode: Age: 79

Recent laryngectomy, therefore cannot speak. Heart condition and walks with walker. Very angry. Mental status questioned by team.

Depressed: Mrs. Walsh: Age: 88

Currently in wheelchair as result of hip fracture and cardiac problems. Widowed within past 2 weeks.

Depressed/Confused: Ms. McKenzie: Age: 74

Variety of physical ailments: moderate to severe memory loss. Reality assessment in question.

Depressed/Angry: Mrs. Borst: Age: 78

Variety of physical ailments which flared up within past 2 months, living in own home. Until then, she'd been very active. Some memory loss: mental status questioned by team.

*The Group Discussion Begins*

| | |
|---|---|
| *Ms. McKenzie:* | (With a charming and marked Glaswegian burr) "Now, could you tell me what this meeting is all about?" |
| *Dr. S.:* | "Ms. McKenzie, you asked the same question the last 2 times you were here. We'll tell you again— try to remember." |
| *Ms. McKenzie:* | "Me? I was never here before. I never saw any of these people before!" |
| *Mrs. Topak:* | "Don't you remember me? You told us all about Glasgow and how much you loved it." |
| *Ms. McKenzie:* | (With a look of surprise). "Tell me, what is this meeting all about?." |
| *Mrs. Freed:* | (With a slight Austrian accent). "Dr. Saul explained the last 2 times, that we meet together to learn about this place and to ask questions. Why can't you remember?" |
| *Ms. McKenzie:* | "I was never here before." (The others sigh and Mrs. Freed takes the focus away from Ms. McKenzie)." |
| *Mrs. Freed:* | "We have a new lady here. What is your name dear?" |
| *Mrs. Walsh:* | "My name is Jean Walsh. I've been very ill. My husband died you know, and I'm upset." |

Note: Mrs. Walsh's husband died 2 weeks ago, and we were waiting for her to be ready for group. It was our intention to help her deal with her loss, and she brought it out at once.''

| | |
|---|---|
| *Dr. S.:* | "Would you want to talk to us about it? What happened?" |
| *Mrs. Walsh:* | "We were living together in our apartment until 2 months ago. Then I got too weak to cook and clean. My husband had a heart attack and my niece and her husband took us to the hospital." |
| *Dr. S.:* | "Did you both become ill at the same time?" |
| *Mrs. Walsh:* | "Yes, and it was very frightening." |
| *Mrs. Freed:* | "Could the lady talk a little louder, I don't hear so well." |
| *Mrs. Walsh:* | "That is one of my troubles. I talk softly. My husband always complains about it." (Note the use of the present tense). |
| *Dr. S.:* | "Try to speak a little louder. And then what happened?" |
| *Mrs. Walsh:* | "Well, our doctor and the social worker convinced us that we could not manage in our apartment. My niece found this place and we were brought in together. We were on the same floor, but not in the same room. But they gave me a private room and my husband came to be with me most of the time." |
| *Mrs. Topak:* | "At least you could see him every day." |
| *Mrs. Walsh:* | "Yes. If only I could have seen him once more before he went." (She weeps). "I miss him so much." |
| *Mrs. Freed to Mrs. Walsh:* | "I know just how you feel. It's terrible to lose a man you loved so much. I remember how shocked I was. It was like a bad dream. He was much older than me—15 years. It took a long time before I came to myself." |

| | |
|---|---|
| *Mrs. Topak:* | "The same with me. My husband and I worked together for many years. Then suddenly he was gone, and I was all alone. It took a long time before I was able to work again." |
| *Ms. McKenzie:* | "Not me. I never had any problems. I never got married in the 1st place." (She giggles). |
| *Mrs. Borst::* | (In anger, gets up and says). "Enough of this. I don't belong here. These people are garbage. They are all lunatics. I'm an intelligent woman. My father was a famous lawyer—and a shoemaker. I don't belong with these people." (She storms out of the room). |
| *Mrs. Topak:* | "She always does that. She is very angry at her children. She always tells us how rich they are and what beautiful houses they have." |
| *Dr. S.:* | "Did she hurt your feelings?." |
| *Mrs. Freed:* | "No. I feel sorry for her. So much anger." |
| *Dr. S.:* | "Mrs. Walsh, does any of this help you?" |
| *Mrs. Walsh:* | "Yes a little. It's good to know that you are not alone and that there are good people who understand how you feel." (She turns to Mrs. Freed and Mrs. Topak who non-verbally acknowledges her thanks). I'm expecting my niece and my lawyer. Will they know where I am?" |
| *Dr. S.:* | "Yes, we informed the floor nurse, and she promised to come for you when they show up." |

At this point, as if on cue, the floor aide comes in to announce that Mrs. Walsh's visitors have arrived and wheels her away.

| | |
|---|---|
| *Mrs. Freed:* | "She is still going to have a sad time. I'm sorry for her—but yet she had her husband up until now. I've been a widow for many many years." |
| *Mrs. Topak:* | "Me too." |

At this point, Mr. Goode, who listened attentively and nonverbally expressed his feelings with motions, facial expressions and signs—which were very clear to all, stands up.

| | |
|---|---|
| *Dr. S.:* | "Mr. Goode, do you want to say something?" |
| *Mr. Goode:* | He shakes his head, "yes." He then does a charade with his hands, face and body—which communicates to us that he wants to leave. |

I am pleased that he stayed as long as he did (20 minutes) as in the past he could tolerate only 5 or 10 minutes.

| | |
|---|---|
| *Dr. S.:* | "Mr. Goode. We would like you to stay. But you know you are free to leave when ever you wish." |
| *Mr. Goode:* | Gesticulates thanks to all. Says good-bye and leaves. |
| *Dr. S.:* | "Well, I guess we are losing some of our members today." |
| *Mrs. Freed:* | "It's not you, Dr. Saul, we like you. But it's very hard to be here." |
| *Dr. S.:* | "What do you mean? Could you explain it better?" |
| *Mrs. Freed:* | "Well, when you are used to leading your own life and doing what you want to do, when you want to do it—it is very hard to have to adjust to schedules." |
| *Dr. S.:* | "What is the most difficult thing for you?" |
| *Mrs. Freed:* | "To have to ask some one to do something for me. I'm upset that I cannot do it myself." |
| *Ms. McKenzie:* | "How much longer is this group going to last? What time is it? I have to go home and make supper for my brother." |

Actually Ms. McKenzie has been in the SNF for several months. She came from a hospital where she'd been a patient for 1½ months. Her brother has been dead for 5 years. A staff team has decided a "matter of fact" approach should be used with her.

| | |
|---|---|
| *Dr. S.:* | "Ms. McKenzie, you live here." |
| *Ms. McKenzie:* | "Here, where is here?" |

| | |
|---|---|
| *Dr. S.:* | "Here is this home. Your room is 315. You have your meals here and you sleep here." |
| *Ms. McKenzie:* | Listens, gets very serious and angrily replies: "This is not so. I came here this morning and I'm going home this afternoon to cook supper for my brother. I am not going to stay here and listen to your lies." She gets up and leaves the room. |
| *Dr. S.:* | "Well, that leaves two people." |
| *Mrs. Topak to Mrs. Freed:* | "Where did you come from before the United States?" |
| *Mrs. Freed:* | "I was born in Vienna and lived there until Hitler." |
| *Mrs. Topak:* | "I too came from Vienna." |

The two women look at each other.

| | |
|---|---|
| *Dr. S.:* | "Where did you live in Vienna?" |

Both women locate different areas, but both know where they are.

| | |
|---|---|
| *Mrs. Topak:* | "Where do you sit in the dining room?" |
| *Mrs. Freed:* | "At table #8." |
| *Mrs. Topak:* | "Good, I'll come to you and we can talk after supper. |

The two women begin to talk in German, delighted to have found one another.

The session has ended after one hour of meeting. Mrs. Topak wheels Mrs. Freed to the O.T. room where they continue their new found relationship.

### Epilogue

My notes at the close of this session read:

1. Mrs. Freed's depression seems to be the main cause for her confusion. During the group sessions, as she became more at ease, and as Mrs. Tapok reached out to her, though still depressed—her confusion lifted. Thus she reminds Ms. McKenzie about past (last 2 sessions) conversation-recent memory: and related to Mrs. Topak's discussion about Vienna (past memory).

Mrs. Freed shows ability to function on an increasingly healthy intellectual level and should be involved in as many suitable intellectual activities as possible. Her new relationship with Mrs. Topak should be nurtured.

2. In this session, Mrs. Topak's confusion and/or disorientation has all but disappeared. She has evidenced excellent recent memory; past memory; and ability to link incidents together. She reacted rapidly to the appeal to her intellect which is still intact. The opportunity for her to play the caring role (her life time professional role) with Mrs. Freed was an important factor in restoring her identity and bolstering her ego. This relationship should be nurtured, and she should be encouraged to participate in the highest level intellectual activities (i.e. discussions, literature, music, art).

3. Mr. Goode has come to three sessions. Today he stayed longer than at any other one, as he became involved in the interaction. I will try to keep him involved. However, at this point it would seem that his problem is not loss of intellectual functioning—he obviously is intact. His inability to speak, the frustration it seems to incur; the shame he feels over this verbal and physical deformity—make it extremely uncomfortable for him. Past history indicates he was always a "loner." He does have a companion hired by his family. In light of this we may help him most by offering him activities—but not pressing him for participation. He may need more time to "grieve" his loss.

Staff should give him opportunities to control his life and activities; offer a range of relationships and one-to-one experiences. The group will always remain open to him should he choose to return.

4. We were very concerned for *Mrs. Walsh* as she had refused to participate in the 1st two sessions. We did not know how she would react to today's meeting. The people in the group knew via the informal channels of communication, re: her husband's death. They were ready to deal with it, but how to introduce it? Obviously Mrs. W. was ready to deal with it herself, and she introduced herself and put her problem on the table. The group reacted to the leader's direction as he encouraged Mrs. Walsh to share her feelings. They extended their sympathy and shared their experiences with widowhood. The therapeutic effect for Mrs. Walsh is evident. Though as a rule, people are not withdrawn from the group while it is in session an exception was made for Mrs. Walsh—thus reinforcing our caring attitude.

5. Ms. McKenzie's organic involvement is clear as the meeting progresses. The interdisciplinary notes indicate that though we have noted no improvement, there does not seem to be any marked deterioration either. This would indicate that our combined efforts may have retarded the deteriorative process and should be continued.

Staff should continue its "matter of fact" approach; offering direct statements of her realities in an appropriate and compassionate manner.

6. Mrs. Borst presents a picture of a furiously angry depressed woman. Notes from family meetings indicate that she has always been an insensitive and haughty person—her medical history includes cardiac heart failure, syncope, delusions of grandeur episodes, unprovoked outbursts of anger. The combination of physical and mental illness, coupled with her current reactive depression, suggests that staff be very careful of the possibility that she may strike out, possibly physically hurting another frail resident. We shall continue to appeal to her intellect and her rationality.

## Follow-Up Note

(a) A special German speaking group involving Mrs. Freed, Mrs. Topak and other highly intellectual residents was formed. The results were gratifying.

(b) Mrs. Borst—after two months—had a full scale psychotic incident and had to be treated in a psychiatric hospital.

# USES OF GROUPS WITH RELATIVES
# OF DEPENDENT OLDER ADULTS

Margaret E. Hartford
Rebecca Parsons

ABSTRACT. This paper reviews and analyzes work with several small groups of relatives of older adults who have increased dependency problems due to physical frailty, diagnosed brain diseases, disorganization, memory loss, reduced mobility, depression and other physical and mental changes. Content includes: 1) Usefulness of group approaches with peers led by professionals (social workers, social gerontologists, psychologists) for stresses experienced by the care giving relatives; 2) group objectives including; support giving, understanding the older relatives' problems and behaviors, anticipatory planning for inevitable changes, coping, improved interpersonal functioning, and gaining insight to feelings of both the older person and the care giving relative; 3) group processes deliberately used by workers in the creation, convening, maintenance and termination of these groups; 4) repetitive themes of concern expressed by the care givers and their dependent relatives.

## Rationale for the Group

The decision to offer time limited, closed membership groups of people who had an aging dependent relative came as the result of many kinds of requests by people who were seeking assistance in dealing with an older relative. Frequently the request for assistance or understanding ws not for the older relative who was becoming increasingly dependent, or deteriorating, but for the concerned or care taking relative: daughter, son, niece or nephew, brother or sister, spouse or friend. The need was not only for emotional support, but for gaining greater understanding of the processes of aging, for help in planning and direction for future action, for locating resources, for understanding roles and relationships, and for acquiring behavior appropriate in the particular situations. While each request was unique, there were com-

Margaret E. Hartford, PhD, is a Professor of Gerontology and Social Work, Leonard Davis School of Gerontology, University of Southern California. Rebecca Parsons, MSG/MSW, is with the Multi-Purpose Senior Service Project, Jewish Family Services, Los Angeles.

This paper was delivered, in part, at the Conference on Social Work with Groups, Arlington, Texas, November 1980.

© 1983 by The Haworth Press, Inc. All rights reserved.

77

mon or similar themes in each family. Previous life patterns of family relationships, socio-economic status and the current physical and psychological
condition of the dependent relative, made each situation unique, but there
were enough similarities in the feelings and experiences of the concerned
relatives, that a group modality appeared to be useful. All potential participants seemed to need the kinds of assistance which a group could offer.

While word of mouth reports would suggest that many groups of this sort
are offered in mental health, social work, and other counselling services,
an extensive literature search did not produce much written evidence about
relative groups. There were a few articles about groups of adults whose older
relative was in a nursing home or long term care facility. There were reports
of groups of primary caretakers for excessively frail and dependent older
adults with diagnosed mental disorders. But lacking any clear formulation
of group approaches through previous experiences, it was decided to establish
our own approach based on our understanding of the nature of the problems
and group processes, and the orientation of the available leadership; an experienced practitioner and group work educator/gerontologist, and student
trainees in gerontology/social work and gerontology/psychology in their last
semester of professional education. (Margaret E. Hartford, Ph.D., Rebecca
Parsons, MSG/MSW, and Sam Popkin, M.A., a trainee in Clinical Aging
and Psychology).

*Pregroup Planning*

In pregroup planning, account was taken of the influence of the context
which was the Adult Counselling Center of the Andrus Gerontology Center
on the campus of the University of Southern California.

The potential participants were people who had called the Center re-
questing help about an older relative, or were currently receiving individual
counselling at the Center.

An eclectic group approach was used, that is, drawing from various
theoretical orientations as it seemed appropriate for the needs of the participants. Less of an encounter approach or of long term psychotherapy were
used, and more of a supportive, current functioning, reality orientation, dealing with crises as they occurred with some didactic educational approach
to understanding the normal and pathological changes in aging, and with
an emphasis on helping participants cope with and master their current
situations.

The focus of the group was to assess and bring to current awareness
through the group processes, the needs of the individual participants relevant to the pressures they felt about their relatives, to assess and begin to
work on some ways of coping with the tensions and feelings and respon-

sibilities of the concerned and/or care taking relatives about their older relatives; and to develop an understanding of the aging processes, their own and their relatives'; to deal with role changes, and other areas of stress. Attention was given to an examination of current and life long patterns of relationships between older and younger family members to see how these tended to impede or help cope with their current situations. On the basis of their current situations, assessments were made as to anticipated and inevitable changes in the condition of the older person and planning for future courses of action.

From the standpoint of the group, the objective was to establish an atmosphere that would permit and support expression of ambivalent or even resentful feelings about current conditions, responses and relationships, and to offer empathetic responses. The focus was also to support planning and direction for current and future dealing with self and older relative. The development of the group was for support, belonging, mutual aid (without advice giving) and strength which the participant could carry outside of the group, plus practical help in carrying the family support role. To the extent appropriate, group discussion included helping participants to gain some insight to their own feelings and behavior and that of their relatives. From a research standpoint, the purpose of the group was to determine major themes of concern about aging relatives, care taking, and intergenerational relationships.

## Worker Choice

With these goals for the group, certain criteria began to emerge for worker choice and assignment. It should be noted that while the original groups were developed there was also some analysis as to qualities that would be important for the best working relationship with the particular participant population. The worker as a well educated and experienced professional in social work needed a good theoretical and working knowledge of the normal aging processes and pathology in aging including the bodily changes, the emotional and psychological impact of aging on the older person and on relatives, spouses and friends, the symptomatic behaviors of organic brain syndrome, of genuine senility, and reversable pseudo-senility caused by illness, crises, depression, drugs, social isolation or other factors. The physical symptoms, effect of depression on memory, circulatory, respiratory, digestive, and gastrointestional and urinary systems, the bodily and psychological effects of particular drugs; in general basic social gerontological knowledge. The worker also should have worked through or at least worked on his or her own family relationships and feelings about aging to be able to identify with or empathize with both the position and the responses of the care taking person and needs of the older person. In an attitudinal sense this means that the potential worker would have confronted personal attitudes about aging and growing old, and the older population in society, and about middle age since most of the caretaking relatives were middle aged. He/she should have understanding about parent-child relationships, especially as these change throughout life transitions, and understanding of authority, about role functioning and familial responsibility, not to over or under emphasize either. In this area the worker needed to understand also the effect of unresolved family conflicts from adolescence and young adulthood on the establishment of helpful family relationships in the later years when roles and responsibilities shift. Workers also needed a working knowledge of community resources for services for the elderly or access to information and referral services. Workers, of course, needed a good working knowledge and skill in group process in order to facilitate the organization of a group from an aggregate of people who had in common their concern about an older relative, so that the group could become the instrument for learning, helping, supporting, problem solving and growth of the participants. In other words, the worker needed group counselling skills as well as group facilitating skills, and some teaching skills. The workers' teaching skill was necessary for helping participants learn to use the group for their growth, and also for helping participants learn about aging, to bring cognitive content about aging and the diseases of aging. The counselling skills were necessary for helping participants grow in self awareness and learning to work better on the relationships with their dependent relatives and to manage appropriate roles and responsibilities in their families, but also to help participants see the need for their own independent lives so as not to be smothered in their care taking responsibilities.

In some groups we learned that the worker needed to have worked on his/her own attitudes about death and dying as well as feelings and knowledge from a psychological and sociocultural perspective. This was important to assist participants whose relatives were dying or had died. The worker needs knowledge and sense of comfort in grief work, of the various sociocultural ways of dealing with death, as well as the impact of a dying relative on the caretaker and subsequently on the group. The worker needed to understand the behavior of separation and termination of guilt in wishing for the death of an ill relative, and subsequent feelings of loss when the relative dies.

*Time and Size*

In the pregroup phase, decisions were made to offer an eight-session, 1½ hour closed membership group. Size was to range from 6 to 10 depending on availability of participants at the hour set, 1:30–3:30 on a weekday.

Initially the time was set because of availability of staff and space and because the area is safer for travel during daylight. It was determined later that a time after work might be more feasible in the future if a safe location for evening attendance could be located, because the time as set eliminated some working people with older parents, and others had to take off from work or other activities to attend the group. The eight sessions were set with anticipation of the amount of time necessary for the group to go through the phases of group development, and the content that would need to be covered. The time limited approach also gave an opening for escape for those people who were uneasy about the group approach, but could accept a limited number of sessions. Size was determined on the basis of the time/size ratio of participants in relation to the depth of problems and problem focus for each participant (Hartford, 1971).

*Composition*

Intake for the group was done through individual interviews by the cotherapists who were graduate students in gerontology and social work. Potential participants came from referral from case loads of individual counselors in the Adult Counselling Center, or from intake of people who called inquiring about help in managing their relatives.

Initially there was thought of composing a group along a single dimension such as relatives of a person with diagnosed Alzheimers disease or organic brain syndrome, or severe depression. There was also consideration of including only relatives who were the primary care takers, or only persons whose adult relative was institutionalized. But during the intake it became apparent that there were some common and some unique factors in each of these categories, and that a mixed group might prove more beneficial for the participants as they could share with each other some of their different experiences.

*Group Development*

With these criteria one group of six was composed including the following: Two cousins, Faye and Alice, whose mothers were sisters. Alice had given up a job and an apartment in another city to move in with her mother who had become increasingly dependent, confused and unable to maintain herself alone. This daughter had found another part time job. She was seeking some psychological diagnosis or greater depth in understanding of her mother's problems, some help in anticipating her problems ahead, and also some psychological support for herself in the responsibilities she had taken on. The other cousin, Faye, who was herself undertaking some graduate study, was concerned because her mother, who though still able to maintain herself in senior housing, had developed a serious chronic illness, diabetes, and was not taking her medication regularly. Also her mother was becoming increasingly withdrawn, and had dropped some of her volunteer and senior center activities. Faye sought assurance that there was some pill or some other medication that would return her mother to a former mental state of independence. She wanted more cognitive knowledge of aging, denied what she and her mother were experiencing and had some difficulty recognizing her mother's symptoms of depression and deterioration. At the same time she was experiencing some guilt about her feelings and the rejection of responsibility for her mother, which she turned on to her cousin, by suggesting that Alice was being a martyr by moving in with her mother and caring for her. The presence of these two in the group set up a subgroup conflict that the whole group worked on to some degree.

A third participant, George, was a retired man in his 70s whose wife had had a very rapid onset of senile dementia, probably diagnosed as Alzheimers, and whom he had had to place under constant institutional care. He had cared for her as long as he could. However, she had been unable to continue at home because she had become dangerous to herself, to him and to others. He was in individual counselling, dealing with understanding her problem and handling his loneliness and guilt, and anger. His use of the group was to gain better understanding of her illness, to have a place to talk out his concerns, and to gain support. He also contributed to the understanding of others with some insights regarding the feeling of having to take the responsibility for a relative who is deteriorating, making decisions and taking action where the ill person can no longer participate responsibly. This contribution was useful to those facing the same future. He also offered empathy and understanding to the others.

A fourth group member, Celia, was an affluent, sucessfully married society matron, who lived in elegance at the beach with her successful and wealthy husband, teenage children and father-in-law. The father-in-law was a wealthy businessman who had suffered a heart attack and tended to be sedentary but independent, but was somewhat angry and frustrated at his limitations. He had his own suite in the beach house, but generally took his meals with the family. The presenting problem for Celia was her mother, who still lived in the family house, of considerable size, in one of the older sections of the city, with a housekeeper and a driver. In her slight deterioration and confusion and excessively demanding style she was no longer able to keep service personnel very long, consequently according to Celia was suffering from being robbed of money and jewelry and exploited by house-keepers who tended to be transient. She was also constantly demanding of her daughter by telephone, sometimes in the middle of the night. She still maintained her affiliations with downtown clubs, the alumni association of her college, and community activities in which she had previously served on the board. Celia would frequently take her mother to the beach house for overnight or weekends, but she would immediately want to go home. On arrival at home she would want to go back. Celia had attempted to get her mother to move to a condominium, or to one of the elite retirement hotels not far from her present home. This action would mean selling the family home, now of course of considerable value. None of these proposals was acceptable to her mother. Celia, who stated that she was in individual psychiatric therapy, wanted to participate in the group to gain help in how to manage her mother better. She also had a younger sister, Debby who was in business in one of the resort beach towns, and who Celia said, was not assuming any responsibility for her mother. Celia brought her sister Debby to the group sessions twice without any preparation of the worker or other members. Celia said she brought Debby for the group and the worker ''to tell her how to understand mother, and to make her take more responsibility.'' Debby sat quietly in these sessions, except for reinforcing her sisters' description of their mother's demanding behavior.

A fifth member of the group, Elizabeth was the wife and business man, and mother of two college age children, whose mother-in-law was her concern. The mother-in-law had lived in her own house until she had a stroke. When she recovered she moved in with the family because the physician thought she should not live alone. While the home was of adequate size, the college age young people in and out of the house annoyed her. Also she did not maintain her personal hygiene too well, resisted bathing and changing clothes, had some problems with bladder control, seemed lonely and isolated. Elizabeth decided her mother-in-law should be moved into a retirement home. After exploring several such places, a home was chosen and the mother-in-law was moved. It was apparent that the older woman was in no way involved in the decisions about moving. At first she was very angry, and the daughter-in-law felt quite guilty. This was the point at which Elizabeth joined the group. Her concern was that her mother-in-law would become more ill or dependent and could no longer be maintained in the particular setting, which did not have hospital or nursing health care. Her solution for her mother-in-law was to find her a senior center and keep her busy.

Her denial of the actual needs of her mother-in-law, or of anticipating the future were problems to be worked out, plus her own problem of guilt and rejection. She needed a place to talk out these factors. She also had a horror of her own old age and her husband's pending retirement which emerged subtly in the group

A sixth participant, Helen, was a retired professional person who was working as a volunteer and part-time paid worker in a senior nutrition program. Her mother was of concern to her. She too wanted a quick solution for her mother's deterioration and increased dependency. By the time she arrived at the group she had made a decision to provide day care for her mother. Since some of the discussion in the group during the first session she attended was relevant to understanding some of the normal changes of aging in the very old, her response was "I know all of this, I am a gerontologist, I work in a nutrition program and we have had this content in training." Yet her responses or descriptions of her behavior regarding her mother indicated that her understanding did not apply to herself and her mother, and she apparently did not want it to. She dropped out of the group sending a mesaage that she was too busy to attend further. She did not respond to worker's efforts to offer her either individual or group counselling. Apparently the approach of the group came too close to her experience and she was not ready to handle her feelings. The group stabilized at five members.

*Beginnings*

The worker attempted to create an atmosphere of support and reenforcement that encouraged the participants to share their concerns and to support each other. Participants introduced themselves by first names only, and stated the problems that had brought them to the group. They defined their concerns variously; with relatives, with themselves, or with relationships between themselves and their relatives. Some took an intellectual approach of only seeking more knowledge about aging, or wanting to understand senility, or to learn about the availability of resources. As an approach to the beginning phase of the group, the workers encouraged the participants to listen to and support each other to ask questions of each other for further information, and to draw associations from one experience to another. Workers discouraged advice giving and rather attempted to lead the group into a problem solving approach, of listening, analyzing, sharing and caring. From the beginning session, members were inducted into the group process by doing it rather than making the group process explicit. The workers did some instruction by presenting information on understanding the aging processes, on senility and reversible confusion and memory loss, on the nature of the brain diseases such as Alzheimers disease, its control and medication. Although the material was carefully presented with consultation of medical personnel of the Center, some of the participants found the material threatening, especially when they had hoped that a pill had been invented that "would make mother like she was twenty years ago." The workers used the group to help participants to work through some of these feelings and reactions. One of the members whose wife had been institutionalized after several years of his attempts to care for her after she developed Alzheimers disease was particularly helpful in the follow-up discussion of the presentation.

## Progression

Each session was concluded with a summary of content covered during the session and problems worked on by each of the members, and a review of the progress including ways members had supported each other and challenged each other. The group as a whole indicated what they would like to talk about or work on the next session, and individuals stated particular concerns that they had and would work on with their relatives between sessions. Each new session one of the workers gave a brief review of previous session and agenda items set for the current session. These agenda were not always followed, but they did provide continuity from one session to the other. The session usually began with some particular pressing experience a member reported that had occurred during the previous week.

## Process

Alliances formed among most members. They showed interest in each other regarding how various approaches had worked out during the week. They encouraged each other to express frustrations. They gave evidence of gaining greater insight both of themselves and of their relatives in the way they responded. Several recognized that they were being over-protective, and not engaging their older relatives in decisions affecting them. Two of the participants who seemed to be deadlocked in battles for power with their relatives began to show signs of relaxing, not correcting their relatives for accuracy when a person was confused, not blaming the relative for willful negative and controlling behavior. Participants reported that they found themselves in more cooperative and comfortable relationships.

After approximately ¾ of the sessions one of the cousins, Faye, reported that she was dropping out of the group for two reasons. First, her mother had resumed taking her medication, with the assistance of a public health nurse, and had attended the senior center nutrition program again. Faye commented that she guessed that by changing the way she responded to her mother as she had learned in the group, she and her mother were not arguing so much about the medication. Faye said she was enrolled in a class which met at the same time as the group and could not miss anymore sessions. It should be noted also that this withdrawal from the group also followed the session in which one of the workers had discussed some of the physical decrements of aging as it affected the brain behavior and social behavior. He had also been definitive in stating that so far there has been no discovery of a pill that would reverse the aging process. Faye had been notably disappointed that there was no miracle drug. Her cousin Alice did not return the week after, but called to say her car had given out. She also indicated that she had located a job that would prevent her from coming to the last session. The last session was attended by three participants, two of whom indicated that they would like to join another group if it were offered. The third indicated that she would like to become a senior volunteer at the center, and while she wanted to continue contact she did not need any help like the other group members.

*Common Themes*

Several common themes were identified from the initial groups; those having to do with actions taken with relatives, those related to feelings, those dealing with relationships, and those related to knowledge.

One of the major actions that relatives are concerned about is the relocation of a person who becomes too frail or dependent to remain in the original residence alone, or too deteriorated to remain in the community. The issue is around helping the relative to move. In many cases this was the precipitating event that brought the family to the center. An important aspect of this theme is to help the caretaker to understand how difficult relocation can be for the older person. Another aspect is involving the older person in the decision every step of the way. The choice to move the older person into the family home where there are in-laws and may be children of assorted ages, may have greater implications, and carry more responsibility than anticipated. If the relatives are considering moving the older person it is important for families to see that the older relative needs to maintain some sense of control and participation in the decision and the act of moving in order to maintain some sense of self esteem as well as avoiding disorientation that may follow a major move for anyone. Relatives need to anticipate the changes in relationships, pressures, use of family resources both physical and emotional, and the allocation of space that result from the addition of another adult to a household. Roles, responsibilities are also affected. If the choice is to move to an institution, the family also needs to be aware of some of the effects of institutional living after maintaining an independent family household, and to anticipate the changes. Some of the rights and responsibilities of the older person and the families in selecting and monitoring an institutional arrangement also surfaced in the consideration of this theme. This issue was discussed in several sessions and appears to be a common theme of concern to many families.

A second theme involving action, was the engagement of other relatives or secondary care givers. Some of the group members felt "bombarded" by "helpful" suggestions from other relatives, while others felt resentful that others did not help more. Group members frequently found it necessary to learn how to use their relatives or friends more appropriately in care giving, and to relieve themselves of the total responsibility.

A third action related theme was the recognition that there were appropriate times and circumstances for making decisions and taking responsible action when an older relative can no longer manage or at least decide alone. Family members need help in learning that while they make every effort to place the mastery and management in the hands of the older relative, there are times when the older persons may feel deserted, or cannot manage responsibilities, and will become overly anxious if support is not given. The group gives opportunity to role play the feelings around these actions, and to gain some empathy for the feelings of the older relative.

A fourth theme, related to dealing with feelings, that emerged almost constantly, was that of impatience and frustration, especially when a relative is mentally impaired. Not only did the participants need a chance to express their frustration but they frequently needed to accept the fact that it was appropriate and important to plan for some respite care so that they could get some emotional relief. They needed to combine dealing with their feelings with a plan of action that provided a means of getting away from their caregiving responsibility sometimes.

A fifth theme and closely related to the above was a feeling of entrapment in a difficult situation with an increasingly dependent or disoriented older person. Participants with this feeling sought the group as a safe place, and a permissive place to express their anger without fear of criticism or increasing guilt. In this sense the group was used for catharsis, accepted with empathy and understanding.

Expressions or feelings of guilt was a universal theme, regardless of the amount of quality of care given by the person. Members were helped to view their situations and limitations realistically and objectively, and to gain some insight and relief from their guilt, by understanding why they felt that way.

The group process was used to help people to work through their relationships with their relatives with the support of the group, in order to work on their feelings of guilt.

A seventh theme that occurred was the importance of communications and sharing between the members of two generations in the family. When needs change and dependence increases many older people cannot ask for the help that they need because of their belief in independence, their dread of being a bother to someone, or their fear of being taken over and stripped of their autonomy if they ask for, any assistance. Many of the families in the group apparently had a very indirect way of communicating with their relatives, and through the group experience learned to be more direct and to encourage their relatives to be more expressive in their thoughts, opinions and needs.

Closely related to the communication theme, was the theme of interpersonal conflict, that resulted from mutual misperception and response between the relatives of two generations. The group helped the family members to see the roles that they played in perpetuating certain of these conflicts by the way that they responded to each other and to the older relatives. The group helped members to see that while some behavior results from life long patterns, other results from pressure in the current situation, and not necessarily the result of old age. Some of the group members discovered that when they responded differently to their older relatives, and with some understanding of some of the feelings, fears and concerns of the older relatives, this behavior elicited different responses from the relatives. In several instances this behavioral approach taken in the group improved family relationship.

In the realm of knowledge, a major theme was that of understanding the physical and psychological changes in aging, and what is at stake for the older person. This included understanding the emotional response to bodily changes and feelings of loss of status, of friends, of control over self, and coping with these feelings. Basic knowledge of aging, and refuting stereotypes, and misinformation was a theme that ran through every session of the groups.

A final theme closely related to the above was the knowledge of reversible and irreversible losses in brain functioning, in dementias and evidence of what is popularly called senility. Some members associated slow responses and minor memory loss to mental impairment while others were sure that severe dementia could be reversed with a pill. Each group sought cognitive content in this area. These were the major content areas that occurred in the groups, not stimulated by the workers but introduced by the members.

## Conclusion

There appears to be an increasing need for relatives who have a care taking role with older adults to have some assistance with handling their feeling, their realistic planning, their understanding of aging and support for their day to day responsibilities and frustrations. They need help in learning how to take on appropriate roles and care in working through their problems in the caretaking role. People who share these stresses in common, guided by an educated professional who has expertise in group leadership, and in gerontology can be helped to manage their responsibilities more adequately.

The experiences reported here would suggest the participants in groups created for the purpose of helping them work with older relatives evidenced some change in their behavior, their beliefs and attitudes, and grew in their understanding of aging, of their relatives and themselves.

A second conclusion is that workers with such groups need to be skilled in group leadership, in understanding of human behavior from a development standpoint, and a psycho dynamic view of the family and individual, and must be particularly knowledgeable about aging processes as well as attitudes and stereotypes about aging.

With skilled leadership groups can be a most useful and helpful means of providing caretakers of their older relatives to be able to function adequately and appropriately, hopefully to improve the quality of life for older adults and their families.

## BIBLIOGRAPHY

Hartford, Margaret E. Groups in Social Work. New York: Columbia University Press, 1971.
Hartford, Margaret E. Use of Groups in Mental Health of the Elderly, J. Birren and Sloane, Handbook of Mental Health in Aging. Englewood Cliffs: Prentice Hall, 1980.

# GROUP WORK WITH KIN
# AND FRIENDS CARING FOR THE ELDERLY

George Getzel

ABSTRACT. The significant roles of kin and friends in caring for the frail elderly necessitates an extension of group services to this population. The rationale for caregiver groups is developed through an examination of gerontological research. A group program and a practice framework for services to kin and friends are presented. Practice issues in running groups entail profound stresses on families and friends and the worker's ability to face thematic and interactional problems of considerable intensity. Guidelines for intervention are specified to handle phase specific situations in these groups.

## Introduction

To face a frail elderly parent in your middle-age or a declining spouse in the autumnal years of marriage is an encounter which confirms our human frailty. Social workers are increasingly seeing people whose aging relatives overwhelm their capacity to deal with life demands. The wish to care for a beloved relative becomes a painful experience. Very often caregivers feel isolated in their anguish. A group program for family caregivers is an attempt to assist them in discovering the universality of their condition and to find the meaning of the caregiving role which is often misunderstood, denied, and unappreciated in society.

The group work program described in this paper is part of the Natural Support Program of the Community Service Society of New York. N.S.P. includes a range of counselling, respite, information and referral, and advocacy services to relatives and close friends of the community, noninstitutionalized elderly. Groups provide counselling, educational content and social action opportunities to persons who generally are unaware of available options to enhance their caring activities. The needs of caregivers significantly test our skills in new and far-reaching ways.

Group work has played a significant role in helping the aged overcome loneliness and social isolation in community centers and institutional set-

George Getzel, DSW, is an Associate Professor, Hunter College, School of Social Work.

© 1983 by The Haworth Press, Inc. All rights reserved.

tings. Emphasis has been placed on group activities replacing social roles and meeting the special needs of older persons (Kubie and Landau 1954, Vickery 1972, Lowy 1979). While this approach to group work services is valuable for many older persons, attention to informal social supports that are crucial to the well-being of aged in their everyday lives, tends to be overlooked.

Formed or convened groups in senior centers conceptualize provision to the elderly as substitutive, filling gaps in the absence of the support of family, friends and neighbors. A strongly imbedded belief pervades much of professional practice that says that most elderly are bereft of close caring people in their neighborhoods or communities. Social workers, true to a recurrent missionary spirit, frequently see their interventions in isolation from the efforts of others in the interpersonal environment of the aged with some exceptions (Kirschner 1978, Silverman and others, 1977, 1979).

This paper addresses the issues of creating groups that include kin and friends as a means of providing a realistic service approach to the elderly in the community. While this approach cannot be a substitute for needed programs such as home health care and nursing homes, group services to informal caregivers have broad implications for the delivery of long-term care to the frail elderly. The areas described in this paper are the rationale for work with family and friends of the elderly grounded in research, a group service design and its practice framework and an analysis of the issues confronted in groups of caregivers.

### Rationale: Review of Research Findings

Substantial research on informal social supports in the last twenty years attests to the significance of family, friends, neighbors and other non-professionals in sustaining the elderly in their communities. Informal social supports are especially important as the elderly become naturally dependent on others in the last years of life.

Middle aged women and men to a lesser extent  assume major responsibility for physically and mentally impaired elderly parents and other relatives. Aging spouses, husbands and siblings may also provide significant assistance to each other during periods of crisis and incapacitation. Important reciprocal relationships exist between the elderly and their kin, friends and neighbors that provide social contact, crisis management and resources and assistance with the physical and the instrumental tasks of daily living.

Evidence of frequent contact between children and elderly parents is repeatedly identified. Shanas (1979) found that more than half (53%) of older people saw a child on that day or the day prior to the interview; approximately three quarters (77%) had within a week. Only ten percent had not seen a child more than a month before the interview. Cantor (1975) in a survey of the elderly residing in New York City poverty areas found 81 percent of older people with children report seeing them regularly (at least once a week).

Research also indicates a two-dimensional, three-generational flow of emotional material supports. Older parents also continue to provide assistance to their children as long as they have resources to do so (Sussman and Burchinal 1962). Cantor (1975) found that 75 percent of her respondents report helping their children in some manner and 87 percent reported that their children help them. Sixty-eight percent of the elderly received help when ill and the same proportion received significant help from children in routine chores (shopping, meal preparation, visiting doctors, etc.).

Streib (1958) found that the elderly expected their family to help at times of crisis or illness and not to assist them financially. Income maintenance is widely accepted as a governmental non-familial function (Shorr 1960).

With physical decline and economic need, the reciprocity between the elderly persons and relatives shifts. Most often the middle-aged child who is at the height of his/her earning power, becomes vital for the simultaneous dependencies of younger children and older parents. Cantor (1975) found that children did provide more assistance as their parents became more dependent. Children and other relatives (spouses, siblings, grandchildren, etc.) tend to provide care as time and finances permit. The family is used universally to meet long-term care commitments; formal social services are used when kin is not available or when all else fails (Shanas 1975).

Several studies indicate that emotional closeness exists between children and aged parents (Brody 1974, Cantor 1975, Brown 1974). Brown (1974) found that disaffected children visit aged parents as frequently as persons who are satisfied with their relationships with elderly parents.

## The Natural Supports Program

A major effort to explore the use of group work in helping disabled elderly and their families is being tested in the Natural Supports Program (NSP) of the Community Service Society of New York.[1] In 1976 NSP was begun as a time-limited research and demonstration project. After a long history of providing casework, the agency began to reconceptualize the focus of service from the elderly to the kinship network that surround the aged. The actions of NSP are aimed at strengthening the family's long-term activities on behalf of the elderly. Both group work and casework services are made available (Zimmer and Sainer, 1978). Through a model project grant from the Administration on Aging*, beginning in October, 1979, group work services were developed in six communities reflecting a wide range of socio-economic and ethnic populations in New York City.

Group work services are planned with consortia of social agencies, local membership organizations and churches and synagogues. A variety of outreach approaches have been used from large-scale community meetings to discuss "You and Your Aging Parents" to agency-based programs where known caregivers have been invited to small discussion groups led by professionals (Hudis and others, 1977, 78).

Recently, some groups have taken on a self-help orientation with "lay" leadership, and self-help networks are emerging. A citywide network of caregivers from different community grops has began working on social action projects. Among areas of network interests are the education of the public to the needs of family caregivers and the creation of social policies to extend services and to provide economic incentives to caring families (Mellor and others, 1979).

*Practice Framework*

The notion of a continuum of informal social supports developed by Gerald Caplan (1974, p. 5–6) has been very valuable in the development of groups for caregivers. Caplan describes informal social supports as fulfilling specific functions:

> Such support may be of a continuing nature or intermittent and short-term and may be utilized from time to time by the individual in event of an acute need or crisis. Both enduring and short-term supports are likely to consist of three elements: (a) the significant others help the individual mobilize his psychological resources and master his emotional burdens; (b) they share his tasks; and (c) they provide him with extra supplies of money, materials, tools, skills and cognitive guidance to improve this handling of his situation.

Caplan (1974) sees the continuum consisting of kin, friends and neighbors, non-professional community persons, religious denominations, fraternal orders, mutual assistance and self-help groups. Caplan has discovered in a modern idiom, what Petr Kropotkin noted earlier in his classic *Mutual Aid: A Factor of Evolution* (1902, p. 292), "And the need of mutual

*CSS NSP funded in part by grant #2A48A AoA HSSA

aid and support which had lately taken refuge in the narrow circle of the family or the slum neighbors, in the village or the secret union of workers, reasserts itself again, even in our modern society..."

A group work practice framework must accept the simultaneous generalized nature of material, cognitive-emotive and instrumental resources supplied by the informal social support system. Two broad categories of caregivers have been identified as using the NSP groups: (a) the caregiver who as kin or friend currently assumes significant responsibility for the day-to-day well-being of an elderly person in same household or the community and (b) the caregiver who has a limited role but anticipates greater involvement or whose role is limited by geographic distance. Group identification and involvement are greater for the first caregiver type than for the second type. Anticipatory caregivers and caregivers from a distance tend to benefit from a few group sessions with occasional subsequent contact, while current caregivers are more apt to become immersed in the group's activities.

Caregiving, although a choice in most instances for kin and friends, creates considerable emotional stress. Family relations become strongly colored by tensions transmitted between and across generations. Frequently the caregiver believes that her needs are placed on the backburner as she is pressed into service for an impaired parent or spouse.

Silverman and Heyman (1976, p. 39) write:

> But the circumstances of old age are sometimes unhappy. Many old people carry into the late years the personalities that colored their relationships in their earlier years: selfishness, greed, cruelty, bigotry, hostility. And even in the best relationship will inevitably be pain and sadness. It is natural for children to feel these emotions when they watch their parents deteriorate and move every day closer to death.

The typical group member is a fifty to sixty year old daughter with caregiving responsibility for a widowed mother eighty years or older. The caregiver lives near the elderly relative who lives alone. The older person has multiple chronic impairments (poor vision, limited mobility, poor bladder and/or bowel control and some confusion). When the primary caregiver is an older spouse or sibling, both the caregiver and the assisted elderly person may be vulnerable to further illness or impairment and the overwhelming fear of being unavailable to the other.

The focus of caregiver groups is to supplement and reinforce efforts of kin and friends particularly when they are unable to maintain their assistance because of conflicting pressures in the kinship network, changes in the elderly person's health status and fluctuations in the caregiver's physical and emotional capacity to provide help. The small group's mutual aid processes have the potential to support the self-help efforts of kin and friends.

Groups provide the following:

1. information about the aging processes (biological, psychological and social) as they impact on loved ones
2. aid in obtaining resources, entitlements, and benefits to aid their own efforts
3. assistance with interpersonal problems among the caregiver, the elderly and other relatives
4. support for the caregiver who is under pressures and frequently lacks recognition
5. assistance in planning for the elderly in light of their changing condition.

*Practice Issues: Group Illustrations*

Upon examination of the course of caregiving groups, an interventive pattern emerges. While not all phases enumerated are strictly sequential, the themes and interactional characteristics discussed appear regularly in these groups. Examples of the phases come from experiences in different groups.

Phase I—*Setting the conditions by which members are given maximum autonomy in setting group priorities and consolidating their caregiver roles.* During the beginning of the group, the worker allows members to express their multivalent responses to their arduous tasks. The worker suggests possible directions for the group in a tentative, open-ended manner leaving room for members to express their varied concerns.

Heavy caregiving burdens tend to level distinctions of race, ethnicity and social class among members. Solidarity is fostered by the immediate recognition of commonalities. By making maximum allowance for the expression of suppressed reactions to caregiving, the worker communicates his acceptance of members and builds a base for the group's establishing its own direction and style of operation.

The worker credits members' caregiving which is accomplished through their considerable drive and activity. A self-help attitude among members is related to a group as a mutual aid system. In the beginning of the group, attention is often fixed on benefits and entitlements and how to use or obtain them.

An example of the initial phase is seen in excerpts from an inter-racial group of relatives and friends who are caring for their elderly in their neighborhoods.

The worker introduces herself and explains her professional affiliation. The worker suggests that group members include their first names when introducing themselves, thus making the group less formal. Several members nod their agreement... The worker notes that this group developed out of educational lectures on the concerns of relatives and friends. The worker emphasizes that the group is being started to meet their specific needs and it is up to them to determine how they want to use their time together...

Mrs. O., a widow in her 70's caring for her severely disabled 89 year old mother, remarks, "I think it's a good idea to have an ongoing group because your worries never end." Others agree. The worker states that the duration of the group might be discussed... When the worker asks the group how they want to use their time together, Mrs. T. and Mrs. S. discuss that they want to learn about resources and benefits to help the elderly. Mrs. O. responds, "I think these are wonderful ladies for wanting to help"...

Phase 2—*Assisting group members explore together the painful and confounding aspects of their caregiving experience.* Early in group sessions, caregivers reveal in detailed testimonies the nature of their "hands-on" activities on behalf of the elderly. Rich details offer a modest disguise for their long-standing forbearance of painful feelings. Group members begin to legitimize these feelings through giving expressions of support.

...Mrs. O. begins to share her caring situation with the group. Her mother has been living with her several years. For the past three years, her mother has been bedridden. Mrs. O. says she needs help transferring, toileting and feeding her mother. Although her mother's mental faculties are limited, Mrs. O. thinks that her mother recognizes her. Her mother cries when she leaves the house. Mrs. O. gets some help from an aide in the morning and evening.

Mrs. O. then presents a situation of problematic medical care. Her mother's doctor says that the elderly are not legitimately sick but merely suffering from "old age." Therefore, the doctor concludes medical care for the elderly is not really beneficial. Other group members express much anger and frustration at this story... Mrs. O. ends her narrative by saying, "If you can't laugh, it will kill you."

Mrs. R. comments to Mrs. O., "Your attitude is terrific," and bitterly remarks, "The medical people act as if you have no business being old"...

Phase 3—*Clarifying group members' stresses and conflicts as well as creative problem-solving approaches caring for their aged relatives and friends.* It is crucial for the worker to accept the reality that members have independently developed solutions to caregiving problems. The demands of caregiving have challenged the members' resources and resourcefulness. Intermingled with rageful comments, caregivers struggle to identify indicators of their competence and constancy amid descriptions of undependable health and social services.

> The worker finishes distributing a pamphlet on the rights and entitlements of older persons. Mrs. S. notes with intense annoyance that the welfare system is terrible, specifically pointing out the Food Stamp program. Her mother is no longer entitled to stamps because she lives with Mrs. S. Her mother can no longer cook for herself. The group responds with outrage; Mrs. T. says she hates welfare workers' attitude "that you're bugging them." Mrs. S. says, "We got to fight for our rights."

> Mrs. T. mentions that her elderly aunt had diabetes and requires an expensive special diet. The worker asks group members if they have any ideas for saving money in caring for their older relatives. Mrs. L., pointing to Mrs. S. notes, "She's the best for that."

> Mrs. S. tells the group that she uses old towels from neighbors to put under adult diapers to add to their absorbency. Mrs. L. shares information about incontinence pads. Mrs. L. suggests Mrs. S. looks into the use of a catheter for her mother's incontinence. Mrs. S. tells Mrs. L. that catheters cause bladder infections. Mrs. L. responds that she now has a better understanding of incontinence and expresses sadness at her situation...

Phase 4—*Exploring interpersonal frictions among caregivers, the elderly and other family members.* With the deepening of discussion and of group interaction, member reveal previously unacceptable feelings about the heavy demands placed on them by the elderly and the lack of support from relatives and others. Group members' isolation and estrangement become more sharply delineated. At times they displace angry feelings toward the elderly on each other. They do this by minimizing other members' situations in comparison to their own or by making comments which deny the viewpoint of another group member who is asking for their interest or support.

Mrs. T. wonders out loud what she will do if her aunt needs more care. Mrs. S. says, "There comes a time when you can go no more." Mrs. T. says, "She's like a baby. They occupy your time, you get tired." Mrs. S. says, "There comes a time when you can do no more." Mrs. T. continues, "She's like a baby. They occupy your time. You get tired. Children want you home and they want you there." Mrs. L. also speaks in a sad tone of being extremely tired.

The worker asks the group, "What can you do?" Mrs. O. responds by asking the group, "Did you ever tell them 'no'? Occasionally, I have to say 'no' and walk out of the room. It is not easy. I holler at my dog." Mrs. T. says, "It is tough. It isn't fair. You take care of children. It looks like parents never have any life. It's frustrating."

Mrs. O. remarks, "If you have a husband, there's more trouble. Older relatives should not live with the family." Mrs. L. replied, "That's what I'm facing." She speaks of her husband's unhappiness about the time she spends with her mother. She says, in a manner as if to convince herself, that she will move in with her mother before she has a full blown crisis with her husband.

Mrs. O. quizzically asks if Mrs. L.'s husband "should take it or leave it." Mrs. L. says she would probably choose her mother over her husband...

Phase 5—*Assisting group members explore reactions to each other as caregivers by heightening members' recognition of their feelings and their underlying needs as people.* As intimacy grows in the group, emotions run high. Members are drawn irresistibly into sharing strong feelings about their concerns about other participants. It soon becomes apparent that these reactions are reflections of commonly shared individual problems.

Members begin to discuss that they somehow feel a powerful obligation for the care of the elderly. Questions are obliquely directed to the worker. The tone is intellectual: Is a sense of obligation related to unresolved feelings of anger and guilt? The mood of the groups seems quite intense. The worker does not respond.

Mrs. W. and Mr. J. are quite verbal during this discussion. Finally Mrs. R. says angrily that obligations must end so that the caregiver can start to take care of herself. Mr. J. questions this. Mr. J. asks if her life would be different if her mother died. He then generalizes his question to the group. The group is silent.

Mrs. R., as if she never heard the question, says that she needs to draw a line between her life and her mother's. She is looking at the ceiling as she speaks. Mr. J. seems puzzled. The group is silent.

Mr. J. remarks that sometimes you must make a decision that is painful when there is no better choice. Mrs. R. snaps back accusingly, "We should never hurt old people!" Mr. J. denies that it is his intention. Mrs. R. appears distressed. Mr. J. tries to apologize. The worker asks the group to discuss what just occurred.

Phase 6—*Exploring the ultimate paradox that all caregiving efforts will not prevent the elderly's decline and death.* From time to time, for a moment or longer, group members ponder the painful losses they will encounter in caring for the frail elderly. Frequently, they contemplate their own aging and they experience the fright of loneliness. Although group members are seldom able to sustain these themes for long, the worker must be open to this discussion and not obstruct them with pre-emptive reassurances. The group provides a communal location for members' anticipatory or actual grief reactions.

Mrs. W. slowly and thoughtfully says, "I look at my mother and say to myself, 'you know, I don't think you will cry if she dies.'" Mrs. W. expresses disbelief that she could have such thoughts. She repeats herself with bowed head shaking.

Mr. J., looking down all the while, leans forward, wide-eyed and with much vigor comments, "Sometimes I get so angry when I talk to my mother. I even hang up on her." He adds angrily, "Sometimes you just got to cut off conversation. It can be the best thing you can do."

The group is silent. Mrs. W. murmurs, "I know." Mrs. W. says softly, "I think to myself—'Is this the way I'm going to be when I get old? Will I sit hours looking at the window, complaining?'" She looks down. She seems so sad.

Mr. J. says with great energy as if to fill a void, "No, I don't think so. Look, just like our mothers are the same people, so will we be the same. I have interests, hobbies." Mr. J. diverts Mrs. W. into a discussion of her avocational interests...

## Implications

In the approaching decades the innovative capacities of all professions will be tested in responding to the long-term care needs of increasing numbers of older persons living beyond the age of seventy-five. Kin and friends, primary service providers to the aged, will be called on to fill an important function which other societal institutions accomplish in a limited and halting fashion. Social workers working with groups of caregiving kin and friends are devising a program that strengthens the most significant practical long-term care option available to the elderly.

These groups give important emotional support to persons who engage in very valuable activities for which all citizens benefit. The recognition of the caregiving function on interpersonal level occurs in groups. As group members "come out" as acknowledged caregivers, they give the public world a heightened sense of the tasks most of us will undertake on behalf of loved ones and the care that some of us may receive in the last years of our lives.

In a profound sense, these groups are a developmental as well as professional challenge to the worker. The nature of practice in caregiver groups must be tested in a variety of settings—family agencies, hospitals, senior citizen centers, community mental health program and so forth. Social workers with groups have a significant opportunity to extend the boundaries of service delivery to the elderly by testing the efficacy of the approach.

## REFERENCES

1. Brody, E. M., "Aging and Family Personality, " *Family Process* (13), 1974, pp. 23–37.

2. Brown, A. S., "Satisfying Relationships for the Elderly and Their Patterns of Management," *Gerontologist*, (14), 1974, pp. 256–258.

3. Cantor, Marjorie, "Life Space and the Social Support System in Old Age," *Gerontologist*, (15), 1975, pp. 23–24.

4. Caplan, Gerald, *Support Systems and Community Mental Health*, New York: Behavioral Publications, 1974.

5. Hudis, I. E., Zimmer, A. H., Sainer, J. S., and Fulchon, C., "A Group Program for Families of the Aging: A Service Strategy for Strengthening Natural Supports." Paper presented at the thirtieth Annual Scientific Meeting, Gerontological Society, San Francisco, November, 1977.

6. Lowy, Louis, *Social Work with the Aging*, New York: Harper and Row, 1979, pp. 299–357.

7. Kirshner, C., "The Aging Family in Crisis: A Problem of Living," *Social Casework*, (60), 1979, pp. 209–216.

8. Kropotkin, P., *Mutual Aid: A Factor of Evolution*, Boston: Extending Horizon Books, 1902, republished, undated.

9. Kubie, S. and Laudau, G., *Group Work with the Aged*, New York: International Universities Press, 1953.

10. Mellor, M. J., Rzetelny, H., and Hudis, I., "Self-Help for Caregivers to the aged, " paper presented at the First Annual Social Work with Groups Conference, Cleveland, Ohio, December, 1979.

11. Shanas, E., "The Family as a Social System in Old Age," *Gerontologist*, (19), 1979, pp. 169–174.

12. Shorr, A., *Filial Responsibility and the Modern American Family*, Social Security Administration, Washington, D.C., 1960.

13. Silverman, A. G., Kahn, A. G., and Anderson, G. H., "A Model for Working with Multi-Generational Families,"*Social Casework*, (15), 1977, pp. 131–135.

14. Silverman, A. G., and Brahce, C. I., "As Your Parent Grows Older: An Interventive Model," *Journal of Gerontological Social Work*, (2), 1980, pp. 131–135.

15. Silverstone, B. and Hyman, H. K., *You and Your Aging Parent*, New York: Panthean Press, 1976.

16. Streib, G., "Family Patterns in Retirement," *Journal of Social Issues*, (24), 1958, pp. 46–60.

17. Sussman, M. and Burchinal, L., "Kin Family Network: Unheralded Structure in Current Conceptualization of Family Functioning," *Marriage and Family Living*, (24), 1962, pp. 231–240.

18. Vickery, F. S., *Creative Programming for Older Adults*, New York: Association Press, 1972.

19. Zimmer, A. H., and Sainer, J. S., "Strengthening the Family as an Informal Support for their Aged," paper presented at the thirty-first Annual Scientific Meeting, Gerontological Society, Dallas, Texas, 1978.

# BOOK REVIEW

WORKING WITH THE ELDERLY: GROUP PROCESS AND TECH-
NIQUES. Edited by Irene Mortenson Burnside: *North Scituate, MA.,
Duxbury Press,* 1978, 421 pages.

This volume is a "How To" book designed to help a wide range of personnel understand how to conduct groups with the elderly. It is intended as
a text for the non-professional doing group work and grows out of a desire
to improve the quality of life for the aged. Eleven of the twenty chapters
are written by Irene Mortenson Burnside, the remaining by contributors from
a wide range of disciplines including administrators, and art teacher, family therapists, musicians, nurses, a psychologist, and social workers. All of
the articles conclude with a summary, exercises, references and bibliography.

Part I—*Introduction to Group Work* - includes an historical overview of
group work with the elderly, in addition to the topics of contract, group
membership, problems in leadership and maintenance, and responsibilities
of the preceptor. There seems to be no overriding principle or philosophic
base which relates one chapter to another, so the reader is left with topics
that are discussed as discrete entities. The point is made early in the book
that group work with the elderly is different from other types of group work.
Ms. Burnside suggests that workers in elderly groups need to have a more
directive approach. Moreover, she makes an assumption that many elderly
are preoccupied with loss and death and that a major purpose of the group
is to alleviate such anxiety. This then is the context in which subsequent
material is cast.

The levels of group work with the elderly are delineated as follows: 1)
reality orientation; 2) re-motivation; 3) reminiscing, music, art and poetry,
creative movement, scribotherapy, current events; 4) group psychotherapy:
family therapy.

Part II entitled *Theoretical Concepts Application to Group Work* is a pot-
pourri of information drawing on theorists in group therapy, including
Maurice Linden, Irvin Yalom, and William Schwartz. Much of this material

© 1983 by The Haworth Press, Inc. All rights reserved.

is presented in a useful way. The most significant contribution of this section is the chapter on a *Theoretical Approach to the Use of Reminiscence.*

*The Practice of Social Group Work With the Elderly*—Part III—describes types of institutionalized groups who have benefitted from group experiences; such as, the mentally regressed, reality orientation, and a variety of remotivation groups that utilize music, art, reminiscing, and current events. There is also a brief chapter on working with the family.

The last chapter of the book is specifically pointed to educators involved in in-service training programs. Ideas for curricula and techniques for experiential learning are presented.

In the opinion of the reviewer, this book attempts too much, and has geared itself to too many audiences. The description of groups for the institutionalized elderly is its biggest contribution, and at the same time its biggest shortcoming. Limiting the book to a view about group work with the regressed and impaired elderly denies the value of group work in community settings. The very title of the book is somehow misleading.

A more major flaw in the book is the omission of relating the basic needs of the elderly to the goals of group work. In the presentation of material, the group itself seems to be the goal with little tie-in as to how group work can be used to help older persons, to tap their strengths, to provide areas within the group's life where they can make decisions and take control. Insight into the very needs of the aging is lacking and remains a basic shortcoming.

For the non-professional working in institutionalized settings, parts of the book can be well utilized as a text in providing techniques for groups involved in reality orientation, re-motivation, and reminiscence. However, the educator utilizing this book as a text, must provide additional knowledge about the needs of the population for whom groups are being suggested.

*Celia B. Weisman, DSW*
*Professor*
*Wurzweiler School of Social Work*
*Yeshiva University*

# PROGRAM SAMPLER AND VIDEOTAPES

## PROGRAM SAMPLER

The rich, tremendous range of possibilities for using the group modality is an ever present challenge to the creative practitioner. We present here a few samples of group programs with and for frail elderly people. In addition, several videotapes describing group programs have come to our attention.

Sampler 1: *From Dallas*

A broad range of psychological, physiological and behavioral benefits has been demonstrated with the practice of the Transcendental Meditation Technique in adult populations. Since July of 1980, 12 residents of the Dallas Home for the Jewish Aged have received personal instruction from the consulting psychiatrist, who is also a qualified teacher of the TM technique.

The program of instruction involves introductory and preparatory discussion reviewing the benefits and nature of the technique, personal instruction followed by meetings on the three days following individual instruction of the group of new meditators. Once someone has learned to meditate he/she is instructed to practice 20 minutes twice daily. The entire group of meditators meets every two weeks for 1½ hours to discuss experiences and have a group meditation.

Increased vitality and motivation to participate in other rehabilitation programs, improved auditory acuity, diminished anxiety, enhanced ability to cope with stress, improved personal behavior and increased mobility have been seen in individual residents. All of these are compatible with benefits noted in younger meditators, although this is the first application of the Transcendental Meditation Technique in a longterm care facility.

*Dr. Elliot Snyder*
*Psychiatrist*
*Dallas Home for the Jewish Aged*

© 1983 by The Haworth Press, Inc. All rights reserved.     *105*

Sampler 2: *From Syosset*

The Syosset Senior Day Care Center offered a group called the "Psychology of Every Day Living" on a weekly basis for 10 sessions. The structure and concept was an adaptation of a Title I project which had as its main purpose the creation of interaction between the well functioning elderly and the homebound. Material was to be presented to the well group who would in turn discuss it on a one-to-one basis weekly during visits to the homebound.

We recognized obstacles to the success of this project in our community as described above. The lack of public transportation, combined with our knowledge of the senior population and their previously stated needs led to the approved adaptation of the project in the following manner:

A Title I facility member conducted the group at the Day Care Center (which was interpreted as the "homebound elderly"). The residents of the Senior Housing Development (considered the "well elderly") were invited to join the group at the Center. In an orientation session, randomly chosen partners were arranged, a vote was taken to select the subject to be covered, and a commitment to complete the program was made by each participant. Each week the material to be covered was presented to the group as a whole for half the time and each pair of participants had the balance of the time for discussion and interaction. From the feedback obtained at the end of the programs we assessed that it was a highly successful undertaking. Friends were made, learning had taken place, people communicated on a higher level than before, and had fun as well.

The range of groups offered at the Day Care Center as in the past has included music therapy for the mentally frail, a series on coping with losses, and one on sharing and caring.

*Dorothy Wiess*
*Director*
*Syosset Senior Day Care Center*

Sampler 3: *From Brooklyn*

The Friendship Club of the Blind and Sighted in Boro Park, which has just celebrated its 9th anniversary, is a self-supporting organization sponsored by the Maimonides Community Mental Health Center. Members contribute dues and conduct fund raising events to finance a range of activities.

They provide car service transportation for their members—who are both blind and sighted elderly people residing in the community. They celebrate birthdays and holidays, plan trips and other cultural events. The group offers emotional support to members when they become ill and has also served as a community resource to which patients of the mental health center may be referred, as appropriate. The membership, of almost 80 persons, includes people of varied ethnic backgrounds, e.g., Irish, Swedish, Lebanese, Finnish, Ukranian, Albanian, Canadian, French, Italian, German, Polish, Russian, Norwegian, Armenian, Greek, Hispanic, Jewish, and others. The group prides itself on the compatability of its members despite such ethnic variety, and invites the United Nations to visit in order to learn how to live in peace, friendship and love! The leader is Blanche Brody, CSW.

*Sidney R. Saul, EdD, CSW*
*Coordinator*
*Psychogeriatric Services*
*Maimonides Medical Center*
*CMHC*

## *VIDEOTAPES*

Videotape 1: *Love and Learn*

This tapes depicts a planned program of warm and satisfying visits between nursing home residents (of the Mayfair Nursing Home on Long Island, New York) and preschool children (of the Rosa Lee Young Childhood Center) in organized weekly sessions of intergenerational sharing. This program was designed and directed by Dr. Sonya Rath, Assistant Clinical Professor, Adelphi University Institute of Advanced Psychological Studies. The program is unique in the sense that other grandparenting programs are not designed for adoption by the institutionalized elderly. This project offers the frail elderly a useful, familiar role and provides benefits to both groups of participants.

—By assuming a grandparent role, nursing home residents overcome feelings of isolation and rejection while staying physically active, mentally alert, and emotionally stable;

—The Project helps to normalize the institutional environment for the participants, their families, other residents, and staff;
—Often denied prolonged contact with the elderly because of death, divorce, and geographical dispersion, children receive much needed nuturance as well as experience aging as a natural part of the life cycle.

The ten minute, color videotape entitled LOVE AND LEARN records the program. Following the children from their preschool world to the world of the institutionalized elderly, the video tape flows with the interaction between the children and their "grandmothers." We also see a weekly meeting with the "grandmothers," staff and project director to plan the children's activities and share anxieties, problems and pleasures. Selected "grandmothers" describe what this program has added to their lives. The Director of the Adelphi University Center of Aging, Elain B. Jacks, discusses the experiences of old institutionalized residents, stereotypical atitudes, and the resistance to beginning such a program. A Parent described the positive impact of this program on her son.

*10 minutes, color*
*3/4" U-Matic video cassette*
*Purchase Price: $145 + shipping*
*Rental: $ 60 + shipping*
*Study Guide included*
*Produced by Adelphi Productions, Inc.*

*Videotape 2: "When Did You Know You Were Old?"*

This videotape was produced for the group work courses at the School of Social Work, Rutgers University for teaching group process, techniques of group leadership, and the uses of a group as therapeutic modality with frail elderly people. The tape presents group session #15 of a mental health group in the Kingsbridge Heights Nursing Home in the Bronx. Seven residents of this skilled nursing facility, who had been diagnosed as confused and disoriented upon admission, are shown discussing the question "When did you know you were old?" A tape of the first session of this group would have shown seven individuals at varied levels of intellectual confusion. This session (the fifteenth) reveals the vast distance these people have travelled on the road to a more normal, acceptable level of intellectual functioning and social interaction. The tape demonstrates: group process within a single session; leader use of self; leadership skills; techniques for stimulating memory, thought processes and interaction. It is useful for training students and workers in a variety of disciplines who may wish to utilize the group modality. A verbatim record of a 40 minute session, this tape is neither edited nor censored. The group leader is Dr. Sidney Saul.

> *40 minutes, B&W*
> *3/4" cassette*
> *Available: Department of Instructional TV*
> *Rutgers University, New Brunswick, NJ*

Videotape 3: *"If I Had My Life to Live Over Again"*

This 40 minute videotape, like the one described above, was produced for group work training. It depicts a therapeutic session with a group of deeply depressed woman, all residents at the Kingsbridge Heights Nursing Home, discussing the question "What would you do if you had your life to relive?" The intellectual functioning of the group members ranges from disoriented and confused to very alert. The common denominator is depression. The leader demonstrates techniques utilized in the group setting for easing depression through ego support, social interaction, and stimulating cognitive functioning. The group leader is Dr. Michael Berlin.

> *40 minutes, B&W*
> *3/4" cassette*
> *Available: Department of Instructional TV*
> *Rutgers University, New Brunswick, NJ*

# The Advancement of Social Work with Groups

## Fifth Annual Symposium
## October 20-22, 1983

## The Feedback Loop: Practice to Theory to Practice

**Westin Hotel, Renaissance Center, Detroit, Michigan**

A unique feature of the 1983 Symposium will be a number of sessions related to solving particular practice problems. A series of meetings on each topic will be conducted using a format in which (1) an opening paper will be presented that identifies key issues and raises practice questions; (2) practice-oriented presentations will describe ways of dealing with the problem (workshop sessions may provide further opportunity for participants to engage with the problem and proposed strategies.); (3) theory and research-oriented papers will focus on conceptual issues related to the problem; and (4) a concluding session will identify progress made during the previous sessions and will point to further work that needs to be done.

We shall select the problem areas through categorizing the abstracts received for the Symposium. We consequently urge you to submit proposals related to practice problems and their solutions.

Examples of practice areas and related practice problems in which interest has been expressed include, but are not restricted to:

Developing new groupwork services (e.g., working with non-groupwork oriented administrators and staff; handling organizational resistance to group services.)

Unique problems of open-ended and/or changing membership groups

Groupwork in administrative practice (e.g., the mature staff group; strengthening teamwork in agency settings.)

Social groupwork and family issues

Problems of the unemployed

Empowerment through group participation (e.g., promoting member initiative)

Revitalizing field instruction

Minority status and social groupwork

Reducing violence with groupwork strategies

Groupwork for learning contexts

Gender issues and social groupwork (e.g., unique dilemmas for female leaders)

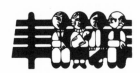

Papers that do not fit the above structure WILL ALSO BE INCLUDED in the program. The overall plan, in addition, includes plenary sessions on topics of concern to all, as well as sessions devoted to issues identified at the 1982 Symposium.

The FIFTH ANNUAL SYMPOSIUM is sponsored jointly by the following groups: Committee for the Advancement of Social Work with Groups, The Journal of Social Work with Groups, Haworth Press, Planning Committee consisting of representatives from agencies and social work programs (graduate and undergraduate) throughout Michigan and from Windsor, Ontario. In cooperation with the University of Michigan Extension Service.

# Call for Abstracts and Papers

Abstracts of papers or brief descriptions of presentations (workshops, media presentations, simulations, etc.) are to be submitted no later than **March 30, 1983.** They should be 250-500 words long and include a statement about main topic and basic premises. Where appropriate, reference should be made to empirical support for premises. Please indicate: (1) what sort of audience participation is intended; (2) length of time desired (min./max.); and (3) whether you are directing your presentation at a particular audience (e.g., new practitioners, teachers of groupwork, etc.)

Notification of Abstract acceptance will be made by **April 30, 1983.** Three copies of completed papers (approximate length of 15 pages) or details of other types of presentations are due on **June 30, 1983.** Acceptance of the abstract guarantees a place on the final program, providing the completed paper or details of other types of presentation is consistent with the approved abstract.

Send abstracts and papers to: Harvey Bertcher, Conference Chairperson, 4060 B Frieze Building, School of Social Work, The University of Michigan, Ann Arbor, Michigan 48109. (313) 763-6571.

For further information contact the University of Michigan Department of Conferences, 412 Maynard Street, Ann Arbor, Michigan 48109. (313) 764-5304.

## The Advancement of Social Work with Groups

Fifth Annual Symposium
October 20-22, 1983

## The Feedback Loop: Practice to Theory To Practice

Westin Hotel, Renaissance Center
Detroit, Michigan